Richard Shaw, MD.

To Hélène as ever. To Johana, Laura, Clémence and their parents, To all my loved ones

The Body and its Pain

Gabriel Burloux

FA^B
Free Association Books

First published in France 2004

Published in the United Kingdom 2005
by Free Association Books
57 Warren Street
London W1T 5NR

English-language translation by Margaret Woods

British Library Cataloguing in Publication Data
A catalogue record for this book is available from the British Library

Produced by Bookchase, London
Printed and bound in the EU

ISBN 1 853437948

ACKNOWLEDGEMENTS

We wish to thank Trevor Brown at Free Association Books for taking on this project; our contributors for making it possible; and Debbie Stewart for her assistance.
Also, love and special thanks for their usual patience to Liza, Jake and Ellie and to Alison and Daniel.

Contents

Introduction

Pain is not a fact. Even the physical pain which could be considered a purely physiological phenomenon proves to be infinitely more complex than we might think: a blow, burn or sting hurts because a neural device allows it to. But what we feel is the fruit of an acquisition.

Pain is an indispensable part of life. Is it pure chance? It is contemporary with the birth of the child and is then just a cry! But that cry is a cry for life. It is an appeal to the adults awaiting it and, without the baby knowing, is already interpreted, already something more than purely physiological. Physiology is also becoming more complex year by year. Neurophysiologists are teaching us things which, strangely enough, deepen the enigma of pain and forge links with what Freud said first and what psychoanalysts have said since on the subject. A dialogue had to develop.

Two reasons have led me to write this book.

The first is internal. After more than twenty-five years of difficult work with patients in chronic pain, I felt a need to do what I had never done before and had never been able to do, despite my efforts: to gather my memories and arrange my thoughts based on the ideas, emotions and feelings I had experienced through my patients. Not to construct a theory, pain cannot be confined in this way, but to bear witness.

It was as a psychoanalyst that I was called upon to deal with chronic pain, but the general practitioner that I had previously been had a contribution to make. It was no help! Except perhaps to give me a better understanding of the *furor sanandi* of somaticians towards pain and their disappointment at the difficulties they encounter, because pain is intractable. At a time when it is much discussed and ever-present, it manages to find its way cleverly between the medicine of the body, which is shocked by its own limits, and the medicine of the mind, which is called in but is reluctant to come to the rescue. Faced with the imposing arsenal of modern medical technology and therapies and the demand for effective cures whipped up by the media, pain - that 'sower of confusion' as J.-B. Pontalis calls it - not only derides and defies but takes advantage by acting like an undeserving old lady who has the temerity to be in fashion.

Medicine is certainly in crisis. It has spawned increasingly complex specialities and techniques but has lost some of the art of treating pain. So it has created a new speciality, that of "algologists" who practise at pain centres and clinics. These institutions have to be approved and their operations are regulated.

This brings me to my second reason. Psychiatrists are wanted, or more precisely their presence is *demanded*, at the multi-disciplinary clinics established by government edict to treat intractable physical pain. But they have to be coaxed, as most have not been trained for it and many of them do not feel committed. As for my analyst colleagues, none of them know why or how they should be faced with a chronic pain sufferer, except of course during the regression phase of treatment. They fish in different waters.

And yet psychoanalysis does incorporate a psychosomatic dimension and its importance and current developments are well known. The so-called Paris School, founded by David,

Fain, Marty and M'Uzan, has gone back to the body to give us a new conception of the body-mind relationship and a heuristic and yet creative understanding of the emergence of somatic lesions through failings of the psyche. But they have had very little to say about pain. They have written more about the absence of mental suffering (alexithymia) in their patients than about pain as a human phenomenon that needs to be treated.

More than a hundred years ago it was through the study of hysteria sufferers and particularly on their pain (mental and psychic) that Freud began the long creative development that led him to invent psychoanalysis. Pain is present in his work from beginning to end, as it was in his life, which possibly explains his preoccupation with it.

This book is divided into three parts:

In the first part, one chapter is devoted to pain in Freud's life and another to pain in his work. His intuitive, rather esoteric works need to be explored as an example and an education. The thoughts that they inspire in us shed a valuable light on the enigma that pain represented for him and remains for us.

The second part of the book is a clinical study from a particular angle- that of pain - of three nosographic categories: hysteria, hypochondria and post-traumatic neurosis. These are three different patterns of trauma and the physical (and of course mental) pain that it can cause. Freud recognised a psychogenic origin in these three nosographic syndromes. They only make the enigma of pain more mysterious. I devote one chapter to them with the main emphasis on the traumatic aspect. There is then a brief discussion on the theme of the after-shock, when the pain occurs as the after-effect of a previous traumatic event which may be recent, distant or even pre-linguistic. We know that Freud thought that a traumatic aetiology was favourable to effective progress of the treatment. My optimism is perhaps more measured, but all pain, whether traumatic, psychogenic or somatic in origin, is by its very nature a traumatic invasion that involves mourning and therefore psychic cathexis and effort.

The role and function of pain in these patients gives them the status of generally applicable prototypes and models. They help us to understand that by resorting to physical pain it is possible to avoid an even more unbearable psychic pain and pain itself then becomes a psychological symptom, a solution or even an attempt at healing.

The pain suffered by victims of torture or desired by perverse masochists sheds a little light and a lot of shade on this question. I felt it necessary to explore these extremes.

The third part covers the theory and practice of psychotherapeutic treatment of pain at a clinic I set up about twenty years ago at the Neurological Hospital in Lyon. It was run entirely by psychoanalysts and its principles and method of operation are described in the appendix.

I shall first introduce the idea of "algetic neurosis" or "algosis", neologisms that I felt compelled to use. Algosis consists of cathexis followed by genuine cultivation of the phenomenon of pain, in the regression that occurs when the body/psyche is invaded by pain, whatever its cause. The algosis is rooted in the most primal regions of our minds and represents a variable capacity among individuals to feel, cathect and tolerate pain. It varies according to the problems, circumstances and experiences of the subjects and is far from being pusillanimous or soft. It has a dual valence:

- Masochistic renewal of the cathexis causes it to take root. It then becomes a chronic disorder similar to that suffered by our patients at the pain clinic.
- Nevertheless it is alive from the beginning. I shall compare the *life* of pain and the hyperactivity which so often precedes it (the psychogenic suffering) with the *death* of the stimulus barriers of psychosomatic patients who have lesions but complain little. Does pain, with cathexis, protect the body? This is what some psychosomatic practitioners are beginning to

> think. I shall try to go more deeply into the question and seek an answer.

Having studied its different functions, I shall also examine the treatment of pain and the changes it forces on the ego. The characteristics of the mental processes of chronic pain sufferers will also be examined, namely regression, painful neo-narcissism and the need to complain. I want to compare the role in these processes of traumatic memories or experiences relived through memory which limit psychic elaboration with the part played by screen memories which pain removes from the psychic scene.

Pain mobilises a large part of the psychic energy. Our job is to help the patient to redistribute it to the previous cathexes, now desertified. The language provides the evidence of development, from the initial stereotypical or repetitive style to a narrative tone that has regained its polysemy. The psychoanalyst has an essential role.

A patient expressed this wonderful sentiment to me after a few months:

"Talking about my life has replaced talking about my pain."

Just talking at first, but then the actual return of life.

All these points will be illustrated by clinical examples.

Freud's pupils and heirs have not followed his lead in exploring pain. Yet at a time when psychoanalysis is questioning if not its future at least the form that it will take at the beginning of the new century, it ought to have much to say about the many problems that pain poses for our society: physical pain or mental pain – Freud never distinguished between the two, except to consider the one as the model for the other Firstly because it is primal and second because it imposes its own economic system. In our troubled modern world the body, after cathexis, is the preferred organ to express the suffering which cannot always express itself in words.

Our society is in crisis and the problem of the response of medicine to patients in pain is just a reflection of this crisis.

It seems as though parents have lost the ability to rear their children to adulthood. Teenagers are obstreperous and iconoclastic, as no doubt they have always been. But they are no longer fully committed to their parents' values, even when revisited by the creativity of a new generation. Everything seems to be going backwards (but is it backwards?) in a world where violent, aggressive and destructive behaviour is gradually taking hold (Bergeret 1984). I quite agree with this quotation from Ph. Jeammet:

> "The scandal created at the beginning of the century by the discovery of the place of infantile sexuality in the processes and structuring of the psychic system corresponds at the end of the century to that other much more tragic but not unconnected scandal of the capacity of human beings to cause each other infinite suffering and to be unable to stop." (Ph. Jeammet, 2000)

Our patients are not the same as those of a century ago and do not express their complaints in the same way. Our technique has developed and I see no reason why we should not return to the body, where it all began. We know that many of these patients discharge in action and behaviour and we treat them. We must also listen to those who discharge in the body. Physical pain is the regressive affect of our time.

Part I

Thinking About Pain

Chapter 1

FACTS AND MYSTERIES ABOUT PAIN

Pain: That extraordinary thing which takes possession of people from the very outset. That makes them long for it to stop and which is never entirely physical or mental. And which has never found words to distinguish between its somatic and its psychic expression, or rather which expresses them both by the same signifiers: suffering, pain, hurt, endurance... And which demonstrates Man's unity: he does not make a distinction; he just knows that he is suffering.

Pain is enigmatic for more than one reason, as we shall see. For one thing, no etymology really defines it. None of the Indo-European or Latin roots from which our language is derived directly expresses the experience of suffering. They refer to working with wood (douleur=dolour from the Indo-European *DEL*), punishment (peine=pain/penalty from the Latin *poena*), evil (mal=malign, from the Latin malus), endurance (souffrance =suffering, from the Latin *suffere*), but not that dreaded sensation which at the start of our lives is just a cry!

The purpose of this short chapter is to present some arguments that are developed in detail later. Pain is generally considered a curse. This is not always the case however, as we shall see when discussing the example of perverse masochists. This can also be seen in the increasingly common trend among the younger generation of marking their bodies in painful ways, akin to the practices once attributed to peoples called primitive or bound to ancient behaviour patterns. But as we shall also see, there exists in human beings an autogenic power of physical pain in addition to tropism towards pain that is clearly linked to masochism. This power plays an important part in some life events. It is both a return and a recourse. As if rediscovery of the old familiar companion has some strange virtue, soothing and above all protective.

Pain in human beings is both a fact, biologically inevitable, and a construction. A hammer blow hurts us in the body, while the loss of a loved one makes us suffer in the mind. We understand this intuitively, or rather we take it for granted and we have to be Freud to wonder why the mourning that we have to go through for a lost object is so painful. True, he had personal reasons for asking himself this question, but we shall see that it has its relevance and it is appropriate to question the world of pain from many different angles so as to penetrate its mystery a little.

J. -B. Pontalis calls it a "sower of confusion" in his article "On pain (psychic)" (1977), which is by far the best text on the subject. He could have written the same article about physical pain without changing anything. We know that Freud often confused the two and it is sometimes difficult to know which he means; he readily takes physical pain as a model for mental pain. Yet who cannot distinguish between the pain of a hammer blow and the pain of grief?

The model might be a simple one: physical invasion of the body and an invasion caused by the affliction of a loss might explain both painful processes. We all function more or less on the basis of this concept. All pain would then be comprehensible sooner or later. It is nothing of the sort, and the reassuring evidence which links cause and effect is not nearly as convincing as we would like. Even if we postulate that one of the pains might somehow overflow into the other due to human uniqueness, the limits of this explanation are soon reached. Pain clinics and centres represent the latest showplace where the eternal mystery of human pain can be displayed to us in its modern expression.

Psychiatrists have been brought into these clinics because the simple model looks more complex, if it exists. But above all because it is often clearly out of place, for example when there is no obvious physical or psychic access to the pain. I am thinking here of hypochondriacs or post-traumatic patients. There is an access door among the latter but it is so small or ancient that it can have no effect, at least not now. The psychiatrist (or psychoanalyst) has also been called in because it is agonising to be faced with violent physical pain that occurs for no obvious reason. It thrusts the sufferer's interlocutor to the heart of what I call the mystery, unarmed and defenceless.

One of the mysterious aspects of chronic pain is that many patients get worse when they are treated in the kind of environment that ought to be reassuring. Their pain increases as if the fact that they are offered scope for expression allows them to intensify the force of their complaints. The sources of this deterioration can combine their effects and interact while remaining hidden from view. They "add to each other" as Freud said in one of his works ("Project for a Scientific Psychology", 1895*a*). Certainly all pain has a genius for rediscovering old wounds, losses and failings because it is a trauma - the first of the traumas - and the waves of repetition can recapture them all. The main thing is to find a meaning for them.

This aptitude that pain has for self-aggravation, within the environment of a relationship established to improve it, gives the impression of an inability or refusal to recover or even a need to suffer which recalls Freud's model of melancholia. There exists a melancholia of the body, impossible mourning for an irremediable and sometimes unknown loss. There are many examples and they do not all belong in the same category. The, often obvious, masochism of these patients is not the only cause, or rather it only represents one side of the coin. This idea of the incurability of pain and its tendency to worsen can be followed throughout Freud's work from manuscript G to *Civilisation and its Discontents*, including the work on melancholia. It is an example of powerful Freudian intuition which is not really brought to a conclusion. It is important because it led me to think long and hard and sparked the desire to write this book. Above all, it is central to the problem.

POWER AND MEANING

Psychotherapy for chronic physical pain would not be possible if patients did not ask themselves, or us, about its power and meaning. All the sensations, perceptions and impressions that we can feel trigger elaborative work of the psyche, which enables us to incorporate them into our stream of consciousness. Pain does not lend itself well to this work – and sometimes not at all - which is why Freud called it a "pseudo instinct", purposeless and therefore with no possibility of satisfaction. We have to consider that we possess what I call "an aptitude for pain". To my mind it is not erogenous; it is a biological fact. As such, it is not cathected and the concept of pain only appears with the increase in a certain level of painful stimulus. Perhaps this is what D. Rosé calls "primal endurance" (1997). This aptitude enables us to experience and accept variations in the intensity of pain up to a certain point. Who can disrupt a system of this kind?

This question introduces the "construction" aspect of pain. In the human species, what we feel at the start of our lives, helplessness, which Freud called *Hilflosigkeit,* has long been translated as "état de détresse" [distressed state]. As we shall see in the next chapter, Freud made a distinction in this distress between anxiety and pain. J. Laplanche's translation: "désaide" [helplessness], which is closer to the

German, places the emphasis on the need for help, which will come from the mother and the parental environment. We can look at it like this: pain (like anxiety) is immediately cathected because it is felt. It requires a countercathexis to be tolerated. We know that to Freud the original repression is a countercathexis. Its quality will depend on the mother, what she can offer and her powers of consolation. Little by little the painful sensations will be labelled; some will be soothed more than others and some will be dreaded, but all in complicity with the mother. Naturally some will always remain, making a particular person afraid of pinpricks, tickling or some other discomfort without being especially wimpish or cowardly. In short, it will go hand in hand with the subject's psychological development.

In contrast (and this is where we shall return to masochism and its imperatives) a child who is not sufficiently enveloped in maternal warmth, gentleness and protection can only cathect painful sensations - and therefore cultivate them because it cannot express them. Pain can become familiar and habitual and the defence mechanisms against it can become repetitive and weak: motor discharges, cries that do not anticipate a response etc. Subversion of pain may occur, as we shall see in detail when discussing hypochondria or post-traumatic neuroses, in very different styles, if we can call them that. In these cases, a painful microspace can be formed which is not really internal because it is not psychized, but not really external either. It is a localized hurt, a place of projection of old agonies and pains, a seed of hypochondria and traumatophilia. Along the way we shall grasp how hard it is to define the physical or psychic nature of these early pains, which are basically the body's responses to psychic distress. Too much power and not enough meaning, and the psyche remains gripped by this distress.

The autoeroticism will then be poor in quality and impaired fantasization will provide little scope for representative and imaginary games. The body, the seat of pain, will also be the seat of stereotypical discharges which will emerge more readily in action, behaviour, repetitive games, violence or simply massive cathexis of reality. The failing internal topographical mechanism will try to find a more reliable one externally, but if that fails there is nothing to counter the pain.

It is now time to start to tackle the subject of violence and destructiveness. J. Bergeret (1984) devoted a large part of his work to this dimension, referred to by Freud, who took so long to exploit it. If we begin with the idea of a child having to be consoled and soothed out of its primal distress, we have to consider what happens when its narcissistic needs are not satisfied. This brings us to Winnicott; not only is there a lack, a deficiency in the development of the subject's ego but the situation is aggravated by the innate human destructive components. They will follow their destiny when the drive is repatriated to the narcissistic ego by transforming the instinct for cruelty into masochism.

PAIN AS HEALING

There is another paradoxical way of discharging this accumulation of excessive suffering, this failure of the quest for meaning and these painful facilitations which have slowly become ingrained over time; that answer is pain itself, pain as an attempt at healing. I am not speaking now of the pain of a bruised body and psyche but of pain resulting from this psychism, a secondarily acquired, psychogenic neo-pain which is typically found in hysteria, hypochondria and traumatic neuroses but can also accompany any of us when the occasion arises, either furtively and erratically or in a more organised and sustained way. That pain can help us turn a corner.

The links with the archaic pain are sometimes but not always obvious. Nevertheless, all pain by its very existence causes the subject suffering it to regress. This regression is temporal and involves rediscovery of the objects of childhood. Finding oneself back in the situation of a child means reoccupying forgotten psychic positions - need for care and mothering, need to complain - which have a defensive function at certain difficult times.

There is therefore a facility for the psyche to create pain. Freud discovered this with his hysteria patients. He understood the function of this pain: to protect the patient from even greater mental pain. The body protects the mind. Like anxiety or certain affects, the pain becomes a psychic symptom. Like the latter, it is held at both ends, a compromise structure and evidence of repression or denial; it is a servant of two masters.

Hysterical conversion is perhaps not the model for the other types of psychogenic pain (hypochondria, traumatic neurosis). We shall see that there has often been very early strong cathexis of a painful sensation which might have been less powerful if the circumstances had been different. It leaves a trace which undergoes a secondary narcissistic over-cathexis and becomes a cardinal symptom.

Yet Freud's idea remains valid, the body and its pain protect against more intense mental suffering. It is understandable that I maintain that in these cases pain is an attempt at healing, or healing itself. It is also understandable why pain sufferers seen by us at the pain clinics get worse when we try to heal them and resist all change. They are hooked on the disorder because it is also a defence and the masochism helps them. This is a form that we analysts know well, a kind of negative therapeutic reaction.

It may seem provocative to say that in these cases pain is a means of healing and is the best thing that can be offered to patients when they are struggling between a need for punishment and a need to suffer, the origins of which are lost in a vague form which combines a demand for care with a need for complaint. These are addressed to us.

I shall add a very important element which does not explain matters but actually deepens the mystery. This is the psychosomatic question, and I refer here to the work of Marty's school and the exciting work of his successors. Among patients described as psychosomatic, the body does not protect the mind; for them we use the terms operative thought, essential depression and shallow preconscious. The hypothesis can equally be advanced that the mind has not protected the body, since this is the theory and discovery of Marty, M'Uzan, Fain and David.

We see very few patients of this kind at our clinics, doubtless because their way of life involving a degree of acceptance of their problems is well supported by somaticians. They suffer in silence. C. Smadja has written a remarkable article on this subject called "The enigma of pain in essential depression" (1999). Over the last twenty years or so I have observed that our patients suffering chronic pain, or at least those I have mentioned above, never somatize. It is as if the pain is again protective. The patients who attend our pain clinics are not psychogenic. Most of them present with physical post-traumatic injuries or the consequences of organic disorders. But they do not have the "psychosomatic profile", they have overcathected the pain, they complain constantly but they do not somatize. I know that psychosomaticians are beginning to agree.

Why does pain cathected in this way protect against somatization? Perhaps by means of considerable regressive possibilities of a particular type which enable a protective maternal authority to be rediscovered or sought. To utter what every small child once uttered: a plaintive cry. "Mummy, it hurts". And the cure-all kiss is also needed.

To whom is this archaic pain of the body addressed? Animals suffer in silence; a cat or dog that feels unwell goes to find its master. The human animal, whose destiny it is to be born dependent, calls for its mother and awaits her response. As time passes the mother fades into the background but not the need of her.

The Mother: the hypochondriac has kept her at the heart of his painful secret; the hysteric has merged her into a violent primal scene, fascinating and inaccessible, alienating her for ever, and has not fully recognised her; and the trauma victim, wounded by the latest vicissitudes of his "demoniacal" destiny, weeps for her absence. All clamour for her and appeal to her when they suffer. An impossible encounter?

ETYMOLOGY AND LINGUISTICS

> *"Nihil agis dolor! Quanquam molestus sis, nunquam confitebor te esse malum."* (Do your worse, pain! Nothing you do will make me admit that you are evil.) Cicero, *Tusculanae disputationes*

Did Indo-Europeans experience pain?

Pain is strange. For some reason men have always had a horror of talking about it and defining the concept. The etymologies of the signifiers that define or denote it indicate a degree of phobia about doing so. I wanted to explore the linguistic genealogy of pain and was surprised to find that the word comes from the branches rather than the root of the tree, so to speak. The idea of pain is not present in the etymological origins of the common words used to express it, at least in our language and those related to it. It only appears after a certain period of evolution. We might well wonder how the Indo-Europeans or the first humans expressed the fact that they were suffering, because it is a mystery: the roots (Indo-European then Sanskrit) which later gave birth to the words meaning pain in the derived daughter languages (Greek and Latin for us) did not contain that concept initially.

I consulted these Indo-European roots and tracked the changes and distortions in word meanings and forms, thinking that their development must have retained some meaningful trace. After all, we can never know our patients' pain, only the words attempting to express it.

The actual word douleur [pain, dolour] comes from an Indo-European (IE) root *DEL-I* which expresses the idea of cutting or splitting. It became the Sanskrit *Dalati*: it bursts. In Greek we find *Dai-Dalos*, to work with skill, and in Latin two words: *Dolare*, to cut wood (hence *Dolabra: Dolabre*, a type of axe) and *Dolere*, to suffer. In French they became firstly: "doloire", a cooper's tool, and secondly "douleur". It is clear that the concept of douleur comes from use of the tool, the no doubt dangerous *Dolabre*, and, by extension, other tools: *lumbos fuste Dolare*, to stroke the back with a stick. *Dolere*, the verb form which is to some degree causative and is doubtless a secondary derivative of *Dolare*, means, strictly speaking: "to be worked by the *Dolabre*" or "to take blows." This means that the most common word used to describe suffering, douleur, originated from a result that was caused by having taken blows. The concept of pain is an etymological accident over time, not the original idea.

I should mention here that the French word "dol" which looks to be closely related to "douleur" has a different etymology and comes from a different root: *DEL*, the root *DEL-III* meaning to aim at (hence the Greek *Dolos*, trap or trick), the Latin *Dolus*, trick, and the French word dol, fraud. The etymology of the word "deuil" [mourning] is uncertain. It may come from a word *Dolus,* which is different from the *Dolus* above, and could be a late verbal noun derived from *Dolere* which originates from the Vulgar Latin of the 3rd century and means emotional pain or distress.

The IE root *BHER-II* means to carry. It gave the Sanskrit *bharami*, the Greek *Phero* and the Latin *Ferre* which all have the same meaning. The Latin *Suffere* (*sub ferre*), to bear or support, became the French "souffrir" (to suffer) which also means to bear (as in: I cannot suffer it). We can see that once again the meaning of pain has deviated from the original sense.

The same is true of the word "peine" [sorrow, same root as 'pain']. The IE root *KwEI-I* means: to make someone pay. Through *KwOINA* it became the Sanskrit *Cayate*, he punishes, the Greek *Poinê*, ransom, and the Latin *Poena*, ransom to be paid for a murder, reparation, vengeance, chastisement, punishment and also suffering. The French word has kept the last two meanings.

The word "mal" comes from the Latin *Malus* which expresses the idea of wickedness and cunning but also of disease, found in words like malice, malignity, malignant, le Malin (the devil), malady and the expression: avoir mal (to hurt or feel ill). Here again it is the wicked who cause the pain.

"Chagrin" and "affliction" do not seem to have an Indo-European root. "Chagrin" probably comes from the Germanic *Gram* (grief), which through *graim* became the Old French graigner then grigner, retaining the same meaning. The word "chat" somehow became merged with the word. As for affliction, it comes directly from the Latin *affligere (ad fligere)*: to deal out blows to.

Two other distant but related signifiers, "détresse" [distress] and "angoisse" [anxiety], have the same remoteness from the primary sense. In both cases the original meaning of the Indo-European roots is associated with the idea of tightening. For "détresse" we have the *IE STREIG*: the idea of stiffness and constraint; the Greek *Stragos*: to express drop by drop; the Latin *Stringere*: to stress, press and *Distringere*: to attach, enchain, hold, prevent; the Vulgar Latin *Districtia*: tight thing; and the French détresse, English distress.

"Angoisse" comes from the IE *AUGH*: to tighten, which through *AMHAH* becomes narrowness, giving the Latin *Angere*, to tighten, strangle, torment, and *Angustiae*, tightening, narrow passage, torment. In Old French the word angoisse meant both: narrowness, defile and anxiety, anger. Note here the change from a very primary affect, anxiety, to another more defensive affect, anger.

All these words have an origin which enables us to understand how they came to mean pain, but we can see that they did not mean this at the beginning. Pain appears as a consequence – of blows received, of vengeance, of chastisement or of wickedness, but not as a basic concept allied to the primitive root. It is impossible not to recognise the child's viewpoint here. That infantile, childlike world where pain is always caused by another, the wicked one, or deserved as a punishment because one has done wrong oneself.

The only exception to this secondary imperative that appears in the development of a language is Greek. The Greek word *Algos* means pain and only pain without any other idea of cause or reason. It has given us *algie* [-algia] as a suffix.

The absence of a separate etymological origin makes me think that for human beings, perhaps since time immemorial - since the Golden Age – the normal state is one without pain. It does not need to be named or conceptualised because it is taken for granted. Therefore there is no reason to define its antonym, the state of pain, which only exists as a consequence. Basically, is this not what we would all like to think?

What grammar tells us

Grammar sheds further light on the psychology of pain, by the manner of expressing it when it is felt. Latin speakers could do it in various ways using the verb *Dolere*, to suffer.

Taking painful eyes as an example: *Doleo oculos* or *Doleo ab oculis* or *Dolent oculi* were the usable forms in Latin. In French this would be rendered: Je souffre les yeux [I suffer the eyes] (accusative), je souffre par les yeux [I suffer from the eyes] (ablative) or les yeux souffrent [the eyes suffer] (nominative). In this last form the suffering organs become the subject and not the object of the pain. Like French, Latin could also use the preposition 'from': *Doleo de aliquo*, I suffer from something. The dative could also be used: *Mihi dolet*, it pains me. This form is still the preferred use in Italian: *Mi duole la testa*, and in Spanish: *Me duele la cabeza*. We would say la tête me *dole* [my head pains me] if the word had survived.

The number of forms available to express pain shows how much difficulty man has in defining it and his need to do so. In French the old word *doloir* (or *dolir* or *douloir*) has disappeared and given way to *souffrir*. We have seen that the root from which it was derived was polyvalent. I wonder why douleur has lost its verb in our language but souffrance has kept it? The Old French word had the advantage of being polysemic because it meant, both to suffer, to complain (*molt se dolent*: many lament), and to cause to suffering: (ce n'est la que me *deult*: that is not what is making me suffer). This shows how far douleur is transitive and can combine the subject and the object, the person or thing that dispenses it and the person who suffers from it. Is there not a Russian proverb that says "the knout handle links the giver with the receiver"?

The polyvalence of this word introduces us to the semantic aspect of the pain signifiers. It is pointless to define the denominative aspect of these signifiers to a human being. He takes them and uses them but whether the words are "Mummy, it hurts!" "I'm hurting" "I'm suffering" or whatever expresses pain, they say everything but never enough. "Words are too narrow for the emotions," said Balint, as they are also for pain. The limits and uselessness of the detailed questionnaires at pain clinics that try to define the quality of what patients are experiencing are quickly exposed. Similarly, any attempt to discern what different connotations, if any, the word suffering brings to the phenomenon of pain that is not encompassed by 'douleur' is just a mind game. Suffering alludes to the experience and pain to the sensation. But some people call pain what others call suffering. The world of the painful affect is a composite and violent vortex. We want our pain to be understood but can only express it. This is why the language provides so many grammatical ways of doing so. None can ever be satisfactory. A person in pain is closer to a cry than to a vocabulary and closer to what I call the primal affects: rage, anger, violence and the psychic or motor discharges that go with them. In the 17th century for example, the word douleur meant the affects accompanying it - irritation, resentment and vexation – in addition to what it expresses today: "Tournez votre douleur contre vos ennemis" [Turn your pain against your enemies] (Racine, *Iphigénie*).

All the same, we can express pain in various ways in our language, as in Latin. For example: My head hurts, my head is making me suffer, is hurting me, or I have a headache. Not to mention all the possibilities offered by the other signifiers in the language which, when used to communicate with another or with oneself, can give the speaker the impression of an illusory control through language and of escaping the intractability of pain, by defining its sensation. But language has its limits and when confronted with the difficult problem of pain, it speaks volumes by its words but much more by its silence. It speaks the unspeakable.

I think that someone who suffers and feels powerless tries to have an influence over his pain. So he speaks. Is it better to be active, to be the subject: *I* suffer, or the passive object: the illness makes *me* suffer? Is it a movement of surrender or stoicism? Or an appeal, a request for help? Like the Latin phrase quoted, all these linguistic forms expressing human suffering look to me like pathetic and moving attempts to fulfil an old desire: to distance and control the old enemy.

Chapter 2

PAIN IN FREUD'S LIFE

In the introduction to his book on Freud's self-analysis, Didier Anzieu makes this comment about the inventor of psychoanalysis:

> "Later he was quite rightly aware of having been a genius in his own field and an ordinary man in the rest of his life." (Anzieu, 1975)

The man of genius can hardly be separated from the ordinary man. Similarly, the autobiographical and self-analytical writings (disseminated in *Letters to Fliess*, *The Interpretation of Dreams*, *The Psychopathology of Everyday Life* etc.) cannot be separated from the theoretical body of his work. In both the life of the ordinary man and the works of genius, we find pain, closely interlinked, a solid presence, functioning as an origin,

How could an analyst avoid being something of a historian and follower of Freud when his works depict the emotional moment of the creation of psychoanalysis around 1895-1900?

Much can be learned by revisiting the familiar environment of his letters to Fliess, where pain is constantly present. For anyone interested in pain, there are two reasons for investigating Freud's life.

The first is that he knew physical pain practically his entire life – from the many ailments he had up until 1923, to the cancer he then developed which eventually took his life. In the first period he behaved towards his friend Fliess like patients at the pain clinics behave with their doctors. You could call him a typical patient. He complains all the time. We can see what meaning pain had for this privileged "patient", what he did and did not make of it and perhaps also what he might have done. Above all we can imagine what psychotherapy is possible with patients in pain.

After the emergence of cancer and therefore pain that would last until his death, Freud stopped complaining. Perhaps he shows us what can become of the pain when there is powerful motivation elsewhere, what he called a diversion.

The second reason is more theoretical and concerns what is conventionally called the enigma of pain. We shall see that the enigma may not be located where it is usually placed and the secret remains. Above all, we shall see that the sudden emergence of Freud's questioning on the subject in his theoretical body of work. Questions that can give the reader fruitful food for thought, guided by Freud's astonishing intuitions, which incidentally he failed to develop. We shall also see that his pessimistic ideas are not necessarily shared.

Through his experience of pain, and the questions it raised in his theory, Freud gives us an example which is to some degree irreplaceable. It gives us a model...not always one to follow.

THE PERIOD OF PHYSICAL PAIN: THE RELATIONSHIP WITH FLIESS

It is amazing to think of the stoicism and courage shown by Freud when he developed cancer of the jaw. It was torture for him and would take his life. Ironically his sensitivity to the minor ailments and illnesses is revealed to us in the works available to us. The list is a long one: bronchitis and disorders of the upper respiratory passages, rhinitis, suppurating sinusitis, migraine (or rather headaches, it appears) colitis, intestinal problems, constipation and frequent indigestion. In 1914 his *Leibarzt* feared a carcinoma and arranged a proctoscopy, which proved negative. "There's nothing wrong this time" said Freud (Schur, 1975, p. 345). Also on the list are boils, anthrax, angina, tonsillitis and a propensity for vaginal problems and fainting; not to mention the physical problems caused by anxiety, particularly the fear of death (*Todesangst*) episodes which often struck him and may also explain the "cardiac" discomfort he so often felt. Freud was haunted by the idea of death. He thought about it every day, which does not necessarily mean that he was afraid of it: "Goodbye, you may never see me again", he used to say when leaving his friends (Jones, t. 3, p. 319).

He superstitiously set dates for his own death and when each one passed he would set another, living a little more comfortably in a protected period until the next deadline. It was 40, then 41 and 42, 51, then 61 and 62 and finally 80½, the date when his father Jacob and brother Emmanuel died. In fact he died in 1939 at the age of 83.

We can say that the various disorders I have just listed are not symbolic symptoms. They are not the somatic expression of a psychic dynamic, the expression of repression. They are not hysterical. They are functional symptoms.

The series of digestive disorders and the anxiety problems remind us of what Freud had seen in the neuroses of the time: immediate transformation of the stimulus into anxiety and physical signs (perhaps into pain) without the participation of the ego which signals the psychic conflict and therefore the neurosis. He recognised neurasthenia in himself. "I have a great gift for complaining", he said one day (E. Jones, t. 1, p. 188). But his complaints did not prevent him being stoical and he could say in reply to E. Jones who sympathised when he had a very bad cold, "It is purely external, the inner being is intact" (*ibid.* p. 187). As we shall see, neither his minor illnesses nor later the pain of his cancer halted his clinical work or hampered his creative powers.

His infectious, respiratory and other problems were perhaps more psychosomatic, as defined by the Paris School. I do not intend to explore this nosographic aspect, it is not my concern. From what we know of Freud, I prefer to look first at what made him the model patient I discussed earlier and second at what made him attempt to understand and analyse his patients, as well as himself.

Because human pain is always addressed to another and the intersubjective is as important as the intrasubjective; it is by opening up to others that it tries to find a meaning. In order to function, Freud needed to relate to a man, a sort of double, narcissistic and homosexual, with whom he could maintain an ambivalent rapport:

> "The intimacy of friendship and hatred of an enemy were always essential to my affective life; I could never do without them and life has often realised my childhood ideal so perfectly that a single person has been both friend and enemy." (Freud, 1900, p. 412)

In the 1890s, that man was Fliess. We shall see how important this idea of a double is in therapy for patients in pain. It is essential to the process of establishing the relationship. Development of the ambivalence which is bound to emerge is the raw material which makes the work possible.

It is to Freud's father, old Jacob, that we have to look for the origin of Freud's difficult relationships with men, who are quickly seen as rivals. "He could love and hate with equal intensity", M. Schur tells us. From Brucke, the master with the fearsome gaze - admired nonetheless - to Ferenczi, the tormented and gifted pupil, secret counsellor and knight-errant, via Breuer, slightly older and still a father figure, to Fliess, the early friend, and then to the pupils – Jung, Rank and all the others - the list of men is a long one.

In his correspondence with Fliess we can observe how ambivalence manifested itself and then grew in Freud during the friendship. The first letters are passionate and even resemble love letters. This was the period when the two very intense and regressive friends exchanged ideas and also their minor woes in a kind of joyous hypochondria, like two adolescents. They shared some of them such as rhinitis, sinusitis and the resultant "migraines" or headaches. Freud spares us no details of the nasal discharges, which did not prevent him from being in very good form. He was in the grip of his epistemological drive, his desire to discover the mystery of "psychology" (this would become: "Project for a Scientific Psychology") and the human soul. We are struck by the enthusiasm with which Freud initially and for quite some time supported the weird and crazy theories of his interlocutor (e.g. that periods regulate the lives of men as well as women, and reflex nasal neurosis). He proposed an interpretation of the psyche that bears no relation to the Freudian theory of intrapsychic conflict and the psychogenic origin of neurosis. His attitude towards Fleiss is one of dependence and even submission.

The correspondence between Fliess and Freud has not all been translated into French, so we cannot tell from the French edition what regression allowed the two men to express their somatic problems in such an unrestrained, not to say lewd, way. Freud did not know it then, but he made Fliess an object of transference, for lack of an analyst, I believe. The great spontaneity of his writing makes his style close in tone to the free association of an analysis session, which eases the censure somewhat and allows easier expression of the unconscious (Schur, p. 61).

The two friends shared some conditions of the sinus and nose, but in their exchanges Fliess, who seems to have borne the pain better, emerges as the one who looked after the other, which reinforced his ascendancy. Although pain and sickness brought them closer, it was these same aspects that began to weaken their friendship. Freud could not really accept Fliess's aetiological explanations for the discomfort he was feeling. In truth, he did not believe half of them. In 1895 he experienced worryingly violent cardiac pains ("Help is needed in these cases", he wrote to his friend) of a type and strength that made him both dread an organic origin and wonder, "if he was suffering from depression based on reason or just hypochondria". Fliess attributed the pain to "periods", "nasal neurosis" and above all to nicotine and told him to stop smoking. Neither on that occasion nor later in life did Freud have the resolve to give up his beloved cigars. And then there was the Emma episode (to which I shall return later) which raised serious doubts in his mind about the theories of Fliess and also his ENT capabilities.

At that time, Freud had no inkling of the possible psychogenesis of his problems or a psychic resolution or solution for his pain. Yet he offered this to his patients. Freud was caught between two interacting imperatives: to talk to a close male friend, a second self with whom he shared everything, and yet to be more detached and distanced in order to assert himself and create.

We must now turn our attention to what we learn about pain from the ambivalent relationship between Freud and Fliess in the 1890-1900 period and how it developed as time passed. How did it compare with the one that patients in chronic pain have with those caring for them? It was marked by regression and the need to be dependent on the one who knows and can therefore cure. Freud expected everything from Fliess. He was eager. He wanted to talk to him, hear his theories about his troubles and formulate his own. It satisfied his need to complain. Do not all chronic pain patients need the same? Regress, formulate theories which are sometimes very odd, compare them with those of a referral agent and talk endlessly about themselves.

This allows two things:

- a different cathexis of the pain, directed and polarized by the fact of the exchange which makes it more familiar and less worrying and tames it slightly, but also gives it body and a certain depth which tends to chronicize it;
- a kind of dilution of the pain within the actual environment of the relationship, which soothes it.

Both phenomena help to keep it at a relatively constant level (which can be called auto-erotic) and regularly maintained because it is always recathected in the exchanges with the other. In the case of Freud and Fliess, the "double" effect is often what might be called dual autoeroticism. This situation is almost an essential part of the treatment of chronic pain sufferers. It is the basis upon which one can work on the empathy that exist and develop the affective and painful cathexes, the risk being that the relationship may deteriorate when the expectations are disappointed. We have seen that this happened with Freud when his cardiac problems and pains began and the situation evolved with less love and increasing hatred until the final definitive break, due essentially to Freud.

For the aggressive valence to override the "tender current", as Freud would say later, there must be some logic: instinctive rebellion against the regression and feeling of dependence on the other – wounded narcissism, disappointment, whatever it may be. Any transferential manifestation draws the pain upwards, psychizes it and enables it to seek a meaning, even if it is not found, and to elaborate in ways other than in purely physical discharge. There is a move from infinite repetition of a physical pain to a pain which discovers possible connections with the old problems, particularly the traumas. Pain that mentalizes and finds in aggression, guilt and the need for mourning some psychic bridges that are potential reorganisers of the present in the light of the past.

Disappointment, resentment, aggression ... Freud felt all these with varying degrees of repression, mingled with contrasting bursts of enthusiasm towards Fliess. But an event occurred that precipitated him into a new dimension of pain.

Remember, he was in the process of inventing psychoanalysis. He wondered whether his own symptoms, both psychic and physical – his "hysterias" as he called them – were the same in miniature as those of his patients. He was interested in their dreams and began studying his own, in short taking himself as the patient, and this was the start of his self-analysis. But his real, "systematic" self-analysis would not begin until later, after his father's death.

It was in this ambivalence that pain, mental or physical (Freud never distinguished between the two) could acquire an equally ambivalent meaning, that of aggression and a sense of guilt. After his father's death he could salute Fliess rather ironically as the "honourable astrologer" and start to show him respect (Schur, p. 139). But he would discover another pain, a mental one associated with guilt. To be precise, the guilt and aggression that motivated him, reasserted and hypercathected in self-analysis, would allow him to distance and improve the symptoms he was experiencing, as if a balance existed between the sufferings of the body and those of the mind.

"MY HEART IS IN THE COFFIN THERE WITH CAESAR!"

This quotation from Shakespeare reverberates like a bolt from the blue in a rather dull letter written to Fliess a year and a half before Jakob's death. The image is one of death but the tone is one of life. Antony addresses Brutus, the murderer of his adoptive father Caesar, before the coffin where Caesar rests. Whenever an emotion or minor psychic event passed through Freud's mind, he liked to quote from one of his favourite authors, especially Goethe or Shakespeare. In this letter Freud champs at the bit, has a presentiment of all the discoveries he will make and grumbles about the neurological drudgery he has to bear. "Pegasus yoked to a plough", he would say later under the same conditions. This quotation, emerging from nowhere, was both a flash of intuition and a premonition. Geberovitch, quoted by A. Aubert (1966, p. 83) rightly saw it as a condensation of Julius, Freud's young dead brother, and Jacob his father. The death of his aged and tired father was predictable, although it did not occur until a year and a half later. Much more unpredictable was the remorse and guilt generated by the intensive psychic and self-analytical effort which Freud then engaged in, and which was preceded by this insight, truly a signal of anxiety to come and the beginnings of a sense of guilt anticipated but not yet experienced.

A few months before his father's death, the distraught Freud has to defend himself against his emotions of anticipated grief. He reacts denying his own suffering:

> "I really believe that these are his last days... The old man's condition does not grieve me. I will allow him his well-deserved rest ... He was an interesting man, basically happy ... I would not want him to suffer a long illness." (Schur, p. 136)

But one of the fateful dates was approaching (40 years old) and forced him to think about his own death. His denial of pain is belied by the disarray that accompanied it, causing him to question his fundamental discovery, the foundation of his theory, nothing more or less than repression and therefore the unconscious! He loses confidence in it:

> "As far as the theory of repression is concerned, I am assailed by certain doubts which your suggestions will perhaps suffice to dissipate, as happened with the question of male and female menstruation in the same individual." (Freud, 1895*b*, p. 150)

Where he once saw a conflict of forces at the heart of psychism, he now sought another explanation: "chemical factors, etc." and "firm physiological ground".

Then came his father's death in October 1896. Freud was astonished by the affects he experienced (letter 49):

> "By one of the obscure paths in the background of the official conscious, the death of my old father has affected me profoundly."

And later on (letter 50):

> "The past is all resurfacing."

He then recounts to Fliess, in a neutral, almost light-hearted style, a "lovely dream" (the dream "You are requested to close your eyes") he had the day after the funeral (at which he arrived late) which he associates with the "sense of guilt, a general tendency among survivors". This sense of guilt, the starting point for his real, systematic self-analysis, would be endured by Freud throughout his life. We know that he would always be astonished by the pain that accompanies mourning and would never complete his mourning for his father. The detailed study on this subject by J. Guillaumin (2000) in "The invention of the death instinct" is essential reading.

THE CONSEQUENCES OF HIS FATHER'S DEATH

Then Freud rallied. The emergence of the past caused by the death would mark a new period for him. After some final neurological work on infantile paralysis, he embarked with almost fanatical enthusiasm and ambition (letter 51) on what he felt would be a work of greatness. Letter 51 is a kind of fevered vision of everything he would create. Letter 52 described the theory of memory and the unconscious, and a year later, letter 71 revealed the discovery of the Oedipus complex. Pegasus had taken flight!

Several currents can be distinguished in his reorganised psyche. First of all, he continued his friendship with Fliess but the relationship developed. More precisely, the two limits of the ambivalence which characterised it were to intensify. On the one hand he had a great need to cling to him, hence the fresh upsurge of protestations of friendship. But on the other hand he felt he had to distance himself from the man, his outrageous theories and the hold that Fliess had over him. At the same time he decathected his physical pain: "I decided to stop having heart problems!" It appears less and less in the letters and the works that were created and Jones was to say much later: "He was not in the habit of discussing his health, except with Ferenczi" (again there is a need for someone to listen to his pain). Freud then embarked on the interpretation of his dreams and the development of his guilt and therefore his aggression. It is important to see that mental pain and physical pain could coexist and even merge in his life. Freud never separated them and we shall see that one could be a defence against the other, a relief, and the reverse is also true.

To Freud, self-analysis is associated with the difficult problem of pain, pain in general, single and irreducible. It is possible that to some extent the pain of mourning repatriated internally what had previously been projected onto the identity screen of the double and experienced physically, the two things not being mutually exclusive. It is also possible that the ambivalence then related much more to the internal object, the dead father. Introjected in this way, the situation could not then be handled or denied in the same way. What was experienced in the body migrated to the psyche and the pain was drawn upwards. Basically we could say that the child Freud had entrusted his body and his symptoms to the parent Fliess and the price he paid was to swallow nonsense, while pursuing his creative work under the doubting but benevolent eye of his friend.

At the crossroads of his autobiographical and theoretical work is *The Interpretation of Dreams*, the founding work of psychoanalysis. Freud published it at his own expense and allows us to participate in the work of his psyche as if we were present. The dominant theme of letter 52 was the memory and the unconscious, categories that he had discovered with the hysterics (reminiscences and repression of incompatible representations). He was still a doctor but already a psychoanalyst, as M. Schneider aptly puts it (1980). The doctor had become a pain specialist with the hysterics. The analyst would take himself as the subject in the pain of his mourning and the genius would embark on an exploration of the unconscious of the ordinary Freud. He dreamed. He remembered.

Seeds of remorse and guilt of the survivor

Like anyone in analysis, he dreamed a great deal and the interpretative work to which he devoted himself, which went much deeper than during the initial self-analysis two years earlier, rekindled his memory. He had spoken of a sense of guilt about his father's death and it took him a year to recall another. Guilt that was associated with another death, that of his young brother Julius who died at six months old of an intestinal infection when Freud was aged seventeen months, a death that he had secretly desired.

> "Everything makes me think that the birth of a brother a year younger than myself aroused wicked thoughts within me ... and his death ... left the seeds of remorse in me." (Freud, 1895*b*, p. 194).

Guilt or the seeds of remorse are likely to produce a deep-rooted anxiety and psychic pain associated with the aggressiveness and wicked thoughts of death. That would be the raw material of Freud's creative work. It is the reason for the interest which makes us attempt to examine the substance and scope of the work and also its limits. Freud was unable to go to the *durch* of his *Arbeit* - to work through to the end - and paradoxically it may have been these limits which allowed sublimation to his written work in *The Invention of Psychoanalysis*, like an unsatisfied trace, a "seed" of creativity, at the price of persistent pain. This gives a better understanding of the role and function played by the physical symptoms and discomfort depicted in the letters to Fliess, by softening the hard limits of the ambivalence through masochism.

> "Pains lend themselves perfectly to providing a passive masochistic goal." (Freud, 1915*b*)

The punitive aspect achieved is paradoxical: it allows and even accentuates the love-hate dichotomy, but covertly because it masks it at the same time. The "amorous" demonstrations - the tender current - which homosexual shame generally restrains between men were no doubt made easier by this. But to cathect masochism meant cathecting the other one, sadism, which Freud only found possible for a certain time. Suffering also meant appealing to the caring and consoling parent. In both cases the revolt was predictable, if only by rejecting dependence, and it was no doubt a history of male rivalry which ended their relationship. This was the concept of bisexuality which Freud borrowed from Fliess without wanting to acknowledge its origins. Hence the argument and the quarrel. As he said himself in letter 75, Freud could not be his own analyst. To be precise, he could analyse, and it is impossible to read The Interpretation of Dreams without amazement and admiration at the acuteness of his internal vision, but he could not overcome his profound conflict or his acute problems of rivalry with men.

This kind of destructive and aggressive element emerges frequently when working with chronic pain sufferers (even if its origin is not homosexual). It is one of the main difficulties that we encounter and the most frequent cause of breakdown between patients and their somatic - or psychiatric - doctors. Everything seems to be going well, the patient is sensible and compliant, but all of a sudden cannot bear it - not his pain, his dependence or the other's authority - and breaks off the relationship.

I do not think that the relationship between Freud and Fliess was a symmetric one and am fully in agreement with César and Sara Botella (1984) who consider that Fliess loved Freud the man more than his thought, "a kind of paring down". In contrast, Freud's homosexual cathexis to Fliess was "a way of making Fliess into a double to serve the development of his thought". They imagine Freud's progress as "oscillating between reassurance through cathexis of the material doubles and the need to break free to create." I believe this need was deeply rooted in the need he had to love a man, to be in his debt or his debtor or to make him a pupil and then pit himself against him. To make him into a rival and triumph over him. The prototype was his father but, as we have seen, the homicidal fantasy had been realised early, perhaps too early, by the death of Julius. If the (psychic) cathexis of Fliess was homoerotic, then, to borrow an expression from J. Bergeret, Freud switched continually from dual autoeroticism to just autoeroticism, creative and fed by the first. These are also frequent relational situations encountered during psychotherapy for patients in pain.

Freud was about ten or twelve when his father told him the story of the fur cap torn from his head and thrown into the mud by a Christian shouting: "Jew, get off the pavement!" Jacob just went to pick up his cap. "I did not think that was very heroic on the part of the big, strong man who had charge of me ..." and Freud in his dissatisfaction replaced this scene with another situation, that of Hannibal, a Semite whose father had made him swear to avenge his treatment by the Romans and with whom he identified. But Freud thought more of asserting himself than avenging his humiliated father. His discoveries, his growing authority and the recognition that accompanied them represented a triumph over that father which left him unappeased because he had to displace him in some way and bring him to life in anyone resembling a rival. He would never be able to rid his mind of that father, weak, submissive and humiliated and therefore contemptible, hated but also loved: "Brothers who murder their father hate him but love him too!" he would say later. Nor could he rid his mind of the guilt-inducing image of his young brother Julius. Many other phantoms continued to haunt him. In the famous dream "Non vixit" all his rivals are there, summoned and present at the meeting: Fleischl, Paneth, Brucke, his nephew John and even Julius. Freud tells us that they are ghosts and we know that in the letter to R. Roland written in 1936 it was again his father, the final ghost, who appeared on the summit of the Acropolis, in the turmoil of memory and confusion that he experienced. Although we again have to admire the penetration of the Freudian analysis, we are astonished by the jubilant affects that he experiences when he finds himself in the position of survivor:

> "How many have I already led to the tomb; I am still alive; I have survived them and keep a place ..."

> "I rejoice in the idea of surviving someone, the idea that I am not dead but he is and I keep a place..." (Freud, 1900, P. 413-414).

There is no reason for two and he has to defend his place. It is no coincidence that the death of Julius Caesar returns to his mind: "Where Brutus lives, Caesar must die."

D. Anzieu (*Self-analysis* t. 2 p. 501) mentions that in 1897 Freud rediscovered some basic memories, but only as representations, whereas in 1898 "it was as affects that these memories returned to feed his dreams". We are touched by Freud's authenticity and honesty and by his perspicacity. The affects he shows us appear crude, full of violence and yet innocent. They show us how far Freud was from introjecting his aggressive instincts and starting to mourn his father. He had understood with the hysterics that recall, with or without affects, was not enough, that the revealed unconscious remains cunning and inventive and introjective elaboration requires different action before it can be initiated.

I want to emphasise this precise point: when does the psychic effort (and affective recall is a mark of this) become or not become operative in the process of change? What enables the affective and repetitive burden on the psyche to change to a different dynamism, open to a representative scope which is more alive, wider and more creative and freer? Freud's extraordinary fecundity, continuously renewing itself and never satisfied, did not prevent part of his psyche being bogged down in a diabolical network of signifiers, disturbing instruments of the soundless music that punctuated his life. As if pain, which is a trauma in itself, had encircled him in a mesh of repetitive, pitiless shapes. Of other ghosts, enigmatic apparitions emerging not like the others in Freud's dreams and psyche but in his life, striking at his body.

THE SIGNIFIERS OF FREUD'S PAIN

The cancer that befell him in 1923 would then take over and tragically satisfy the "need for pain" which he seemed to have and which is so often found in our pain patients.

Bleeding, injections, the jaw and narcotics, these are the strange signifiers that pursued Freud like the Furies. Others are repetitive but trivial, such as the name Joseph. I would not emphasise this aspect, which should be of purely historical interest, if it did not have two other areas of interest.

The first is that these signifiers were accompanied by very powerful and sometimes even violent affects. Freud experienced and talked about these affects, which could extend to pain, but they represented points of resistance to his self-analysis and points of call for the repetition. We have to believe in an element of chance, but if there is a drive towards repetition, it is not due to a diabolical force but is a construction of the psyche within the traumatic problem area. Perhaps it is better to call it Fate (*Schicksal*) as Freud did.

The other interest is clinical. We find in chronic pain sufferers these significant but apparently trivial condensations which attract images, scenes and emotions of the trivialised blow like a black hole. These recur endlessly in the memories, discourse and life of the patients in the form of events. In Freud's case these signifiers are not easy to unblock. They remain interlaced, as mentioned earlier. They cannot be unblocked by the brief reference to them, no doubt too brief for comprehension, but interested readers are referred to the biographical works quoted.

Given the scale of Freud's genius and the scope of his complete works, we cannot help thinking about the man struggling alone and unsuccessfully against his fate, marked by the unending mourning for his father; a father created by the ambitious child that the young Sigmund had been.

The primary area of suffering for Freud was the jaw, which had to be widened at the palate and sinus and would develop cancer in 1924. At the beginning of The Interpretation of Dreams, a childhood accident that took place when he was between two and three years old (probably under two from his article on screen memories (*Neurosis, psychosis and perversion*, p. 120), and the name of a doctor completely forgotten until then "... although a scar on the chin should have reminded me of one of his procedures", returned to his mind when he was analysing a dream:

> "I climbed onto a stepladder in the pantry to reach a titbit... The stepladder overturned and the top hit me behind the lower jaw. I could have lost all my teeth." (Freud, 1900, p. 477)

The doctor (Joseph Pur) stopped the bleeding and inserted three stitches.

Continuing the analysis of the dream, Freud adds:

> " [...] I am discovering the hidden tendency that the dreaded death of my son could satisfy" (*ibid.*)

With the heroine of the famous dream "Irma's injection" we return to the palate, bleeding, injection and even fainting that Freud experienced during the extraction of a long gauze compress that Fliess had "forgotten" and left in the back of the patient's throat during a surgical procedure. Emma poured blood (*Verblutungsszene*, bleeding to death) and it was Freud who turned away, M. Schneider tells us. "We are the strong sex!" she told him when he went back to see her, fortified with brandy. It is extraordinary that the Irma episode condenses all the signifiers. She is known to have supplied Freud with the needle material through a diabolical vision she had had.

Freud, feeling very guilty and consciously refraining from any aggression towards Fliess, used these needles in his dream for an injection. This was no coincidence. He had already felt guilty a few years earlier for recommending that his great friend Fleischl take cocaine to treat the intense pain he was experiencing. This was caused by the many amputations his friend had suffered in his hand following an infection. He was a morphine addict. He became a cocaine addict. Freud helped him until the end of his tormented life and said in his own defence that he had only prescribed cocaine by ingestion, not by injection. And yet he had boasted of these injections in an article which he had erased from his memory. It may be that the topic of injections, and also of narcotics, was associated with feelings of guilt, all the more so because one day he had applied morphine to the eyes of an elderly patient instead of injecting it as he did every day, mistaking it for the eye lotion also used daily.

In short, Freud's guilt fed on everything but preferred certain fuels and signifiers. In the analysis of the dream in which he remembers the stepladder falling and discovers the unconscious desire for death that he feels towards his son at the front, he writes this astonishing sentence:

> " [...] when such a misfortune happens, the intensity of the pain reaches the point of arousing these repressed desires in our unconscious." (Freud, 1900).

This was not the case because it was only a dream and his son was alive. But we can see the germ of the process that he would describe in melancholics. Freud was haunted and pursued by an imaginary guilt fixed on murder. And he could not countercathect his aggression long term in the affability which can be built into the personality, at least where potential rivals were concerned.

To return to the signifiers. The first encounter with the jaw would be followed by another much more tragic one, with cancer, which would cause further bleeding and require numerous injections. *"Blut is ein besonderer Saft"* (M. Schneider, p. 67): Blood is a very strange liquid, he said one day, worried by his own blood loss. In 1917 he suffered a painful swelling of the palate which he disregarded (Schur, p. 372). Then in the Twenties the man who anticipated the possible dates of his death saw those in his circle fall victim to it. Within the space of a few days he lost his friend von Freund and his daughter Sophie, Sunday's child, and two years later his grandson Heinz, Sophie's son. Heinz and his grandfather had been operated on at the same time, the boy for the tonsils and Freud for his cancer (it was the first of the thirty-two operations that he had to suffer). They discussed the progress of their convalescence with each other. Heinz was soon carried off by tuberculosis. Despite everything that Freud had to say about the strangeness of the pain of mourning and his surprise at its existence, he declared that he never recovered from this blow. It was the only time he was ever seen to weep.

Then came the long martyrdom, the local spread of the cancer, radiology or radium therapy, pain, bleeding, sometimes profuse and the metal "monster" that he had to wear all the time that was painful to the point of preventing him speaking. His beloved daughter Anna would have to read her father's words. But nothing stopped Freud. Neither cancer nor the Gestapo nor exile in London nor his ever-growing suffering brought him to the limit of his stoicism. He continued with his clinical work, his written work and his life to the extremes of endurance. Until the final moving phase:

> "Now there is nothing but torture and it no longer has any sense." (Schur, 1975, p. 622)

Max Schur gave him what he had promised – a morphine injection which brought Freud peace and put him to sleep forever.

Chapter 3

PAIN IN HIS WORK

At the end of his life Freud considered his work. He has left us a scientific testament through various writings. Some are optimistic about the future of psychoanalysis and its effectiveness ("Constructions in analysis" for example). Others are more pessimistic ("Analysis terminable and interminable"). In *An Outline of Psychoanalysis* (1938) a year before his death, he envisages among other things two sources of resistance in a patient in analysis: the *need* to be ill and the *need* to suffer. I emphasise the word need because it is powerful. The need to suffer tallies with the last appearance of pain in Freud's work; the first went back to January 1895. It was the work on melancholia (manuscript G). These two dates indicate the persistence of the Freudian preoccupation with the subject of pain. In this chapter I want to weigh this preoccupation, even if not dialectically, against the principle by which the Freudian system functions, that is the pleasure/displeasure principle in which pain has no place. We shall see that to Freud pain is not a displeasure:

> "Suffering has a special quality felt at the same time as displeasure." (1895*b*)

This "special quality" contrasts pain with displeasure insofar as the unpleasant stimulus which causes it can be treated psychically, whichrestores it to the original level. To Freud, the fact that the same does not apply to the pain stimulus gives it a particular characteristic. I think the special quality in question lends itself perfectly to psychotherapy of the analysis type. It is my intention to explain why and how. The point of this chapter is that despite Freud's insistence on pain having a certain incurable aspect, there are arguments in his writings which lead one to think the opposite.

Pain makes such unexpected and impromptu appearances in Freud's work that it is impossible to trace a continuous thread, or recurrent theme running through his important research throughout its development. It is more like a multi-coloured web in which the fibres break off and reappear elsewhere, sometimes in different colours, or disappear completely and are difficult to arrange into an intelligible whole. Beyond what Freud tells us, it is important to note the steadfastness of his preoccupation, the diversity of his angles of attack and the enigmatic persistence of certain themes. One cannot help thinking that the works were written by a man in pain.

A detailed study of Freud's concepts and ideas on pain would not be appropriate in this book. For this I would recommend the study by Annie Aubert (1996), who tackled this difficult task successfully. The historical, chronological path taken by her in her review of the works reveals the difficulties inherent in the phenomenon of pain; at least in the way that Freud had to grapple with it.

I have tried to identify some trains of thought (or rather questions), despite the tangle of the web, despite its heterogeneity, in order to raise the question of the enigma more effectively. Not to disentangle or decipher it but to approach it more closely. Incidentally, Freud himself referred not to the enigma of pain but to the enigma of mourning (and we have seen how difficult it was for him to mourn his father) and of melancholia and masochism (*The enigmatic masochistic tendencies of the ego*, 1920). Yet this enigma does exist, in the ideas developed on the subject by Freud and those of the doctors trying to treat it.

Pain is present throughout Freud's writings and has a very special status. First of all Freud makes little distinction between physical and mental pain. His language uses the same terms to describe them both, as he says in *Inhibitions, Symptoms and Anxiety*. He goes further and declares it to be obvious that the model for mental pain is physical pain. This arguable point is important because it immediately attributes a special character to pain which distinguishes it from anxiety – it is hardly or not at all open to work of psychic resolution. Anxiety could thus discharge into the psyche but not pain. But the situation with grief, the prototype mental pain, does show that this work is possible, melancholia being a very special case, the exception not the rule. Also, melancholia and detachment from the object can be worked through, difficult though this may be, as B. Rosenberg showed in his work on masochism.

On the other hand, it is true that physical pain is less responsive to this process. The aim of this book is to show why and how it can be achieved. It is hard to imagine an isolated somatic pain. The boundaries between the somatic and the psychic are sometimes quite uncertain and physical pain is always mental pain too, the experience of a loss psychically cathected.

Stranger still is the idea that pain has a tendency not only to self-maintenance but also to self-aggravation and therefore to incurability. It is interesting to look more closely at this Freudian pessimism. At first sight it appears justified, but when we look more closely it curiously seems to contain ideas that make it optimistic. We must first consider the texts.

SELF-MAINTENANCE OF PAIN

A few lines in Manuscript G dated January 1895 devoted to melancholia (we are told that it means depression) express one of Freud's strongest ideas – depicted in strong words: internal *bleeding*, aspiration, *impoverishment*, inhibition which has the effect of a *wound* and finally hole. All are signifiers indicating invasion and loss. Two fundamental points can be noted above all:

- The appeal effect exerted on the quantity of stimulus present (this is bleeding causing the impoverishment);
- And already a tiny reference: "see the theory of physical pain" which makes it the paradigm of mental suffering

Mourning and Melancholia (1917) repeats exactly these two points:

> "The melancholic complex behaves like an open *wound attracting* cathexis energies to it from all sides (what we called countercathexis in transference neuroses) and draining the ego to the point of *impoverishing* it completely."

And later, towards the end, comes the celebrated phrase on the need to shed:

> "light on the economic nature firstly of physical pain and then of the psychic pain which is comparable with it."

Freud is always making the same point.

When discussing traumatic neuroses in *Beyond the Pleasure Principle* (1920), Freud considers an idea which would lead to the famous turning point of his theory. The psychic trauma and the break in the stimulus barrier give him the opportunity to re-examine the economic problem of pain in this light. He again takes physical pain as the model, which is not surprising. He defines it as an *invasion* of the stimulus barrier over a limited field. He rediscovers his 1895 outline and reworks it, making it a little more complex but in my opinion, without providing a new solution:

> "Cathectic energy is *summoned* from all sides to provide sufficiently high cathexes of energy in the

> environs of the breach. An 'anticathexis' on a grand scale is set up, for the benefit of which all the other psychical systems are *impoverished* ..." (Freud, 1920)

Freud says that a strongly cathected system is able to accept an additional inflow of energy and transform it into quiescent cathexis, that is to "bind it psychically". The points common to the three texts are: invasion, energy recall and resultant impoverishment. The only point of divergence is in the *Manuscript*, in which recourse to the available energy occurs to make up for the very great loss of stimulus due to the pain. In the other texts it occurs to block the excessive stimulus.

In *Beyond the Pleasure Principle*, pain and traumatic neurosis are defined by comparison with the stimulus barriers: invasion to a limited extent for the former and extensive for the latter. Another common feature is the outpouring of psychic elaboration or his inability to contain or process it. Although Freud's views on trauma alternated - at times pessimistic: "a wound that will never heal but will grow with time" (Fetish objects, *New Journal of Psychoanalysis*, No. 2) and at times optimistic: "There is no doubt that the aetiology of trauma offers by far the most favourable opportunity for analysis" - he leaves us in suspense about pain, as he does about the defence mechanism he invented against it.

It is possible to understand the process of defence, but not to see why it could stop the pain or how it could metabolise in the psyche. The violence of the pain is balanced in some way by the violence of a countercathexis, in a trial of strength which matters more for the quantity of energy it mobilises than for its own qualities. When two forces of equal intensity neutralise each other and freeze in a petrified confrontation, the scene can be long-lasting. The term "bind psychically," recalls another term earlier in the same text: "The patient is fixed psychically in the trauma, so to speak". The countercathexis involved has gathered all the available energy for an occlusive and purely dynamic and quantitative purpose.

The imperative of the force prevails over the possibility of meaning. But could it not be slightly qualitative? Jean Cournut wrote an article in the *New Journal of Psychoanalysis* (No. 39) which perfectly describes these two possibilities of countercathexis. One of pure necessity and urgency and one which, in addition to its defensive qualities, is also capable of giving meaning and opening up to the psyche. Cournut uses the term "narcissistic libidinal overtension".

This point is very important because in one way there is no doubt that this aspect can be observed in chronic pain, frozen in the defensive effort. And yet I dispute it. It is understandable that there is a need for an urgent and occlusive quantity in the face of a stimulus which overflows everything – a counter-force. But must it remain forever as an immovable buttress without finding a meaning? If that were so, there would be no way to influence chronic pain. We shall see in chapter 3 on treatment that we have to question the quality of the original countercathexis which allowed the repression of the same name. That is, what the primal object was able to offer. This brings us back to the question of the mother-baby relationship.

In my view, therefore, Freud does not do in this work, which repeats his old idea, what he had proposed doing in *Mourning and Melancholia*: i.e. resolving the economic problem of physical pain. On the contrary, he retreats into the same catastrophic idea of pain. He expounds a necessary, self-maintained defence mechanism without contemplating any outlet or any means of alleviation of this mechanism, which appears unstoppable. In short, Freud leaves us with impoverishment of the psyche, fierce combat and a frozen situation. Worse still, even darker ideas were to appear in other works.

SELF-AGGRAVATION OF PAIN

"Project for a Scientific Psychology" is a work which we know was written at least partly in a mood of creative enthusiasm that Freud would soon abandon:

> "The state of mind in which I conceived psychology is now alien to me." (Freud, 1895)

It is an inspired work which discusses the question of pain in three very short but very dense chapters (6, 11, 12).

In the first, headed "Pain", it is presented as a phenomenon capable of thwarting a *biological* type organisation[1]. It therefore involves an actual pain, defined by its results which produce a facilitation: "irruption of large quantities", "increases in quantity", "irruption of excessive quantities". Then comes the famous quotation:

> "It is certain that pain leaves behind it permanent facilitations in ø like a streak of lightning." (*ibid.*)

We can see the origins of the idea that pain is possibly definitive and incurable. This is a familiar idea to Freud and can often be found elsewhere, for example in the chapter on suffering, the most insistent on this point.

Chapter 12, headed "The experience of suffering considered as" is the return to memory of what caused the pain. That is, when the mnestic image of the object generating suffering is recathected due to new perceptions. This produces "something akin to suffering" and a need for discharge. Freud has a problem. The neurones he has imagined to explain the mental functioning, ö, ø and ù, are not sufficient to describe this experience of suffering. He gets help from secretor neurones, invented for the situation and called key neurones. It is significant that he makes a Freudian slip by calling them motors (doubtless out of nostalgia for a simpler motor discharge). When excessive quantities have made a breach, these key neurones are stimulated by the *memory* of the pain. But far from bringing about a discharge,

1 I have italicised the word biological because Freud does not specify whether the pain he is referring to is somatic or psychological. In this case he again seems to combine both aspects.

they *add* them through certain byways by means of secretion[1]. Here we have a defence which aggravates the situation! The ego in pain defends itself badly.

> "The experience of pain supplies excellent facilitations between the mnestic image of the hostile object and these key neurones." (Freud, 1950, p. 339)

Freud refers her to "a surprising but essential hypothesis".

Pain does not have a separate entry in the *Vocabulary of Psychoanalysis* by Laplanche and Pontalis, but it appears in the article "Defence" on the very subject of the experience of suffering. The authors stress its paradoxical aspect. I quote:

> "Why would the nervous system *repeat* to the extent of *hallucinating* a pain which is defined by an increase in load if the function of the system is to avoid any increase in tension?"[2]

One might answer: because of masochism, but I think this would be too hasty. Production of pain is not necessarily enjoyment of pain. In any case, Laplanche and Pontalis prefer to see it as a metaphor, based on the model of physical pain, "of the internal aggression which the instinct represents for the ego" and refer later to "that pain which anxiety is for the ego".

Could this be anxiety? Pain has its specificity. Freud is careful to differentiate it from anxiety and also from displeasure[3]. Pain, like trauma, is defined as a breach of the stimulus barrier and an absence of psychic preparation produced by anxiety. The anxiety is associated with the expectation; it is anxiety about something. It has no object. When it has found one, its name is replaced by the word fear, says Freud in *Inhibition, Symptom and Anxiety* (1926). But Laplanche and Pontalis are right to examine this paradoxical

1 It is Freud who highlights the two words; we are rightly surprised by the translation of the second word but realise that it refers to worsening.

2 My italics

3 He refers two or three times to the "displeasure of pain" but descriptively. It is not the displeasure dependent on pleasure, the two entities which make the Freudian principle function.

defence process, which is situated beyond the pleasure principle and brings us back to a recurrent difficulty in Freud on the subject of pain.

Incidentally, at the end of "Project for a Scientific Psychology" is he still remembering his "surprising but essential hypothesis"? He speaks (p. 368) of a "painful experience generating displeasure" and the defence mechanism set up by a "cathected" ego. He shows how the ego, thanks to the attention, "with copious lateral cathexes", will reduce the quantity of displeasure generated and how it will act as a warning signal. We are already in the realm of the anxiety signal rediscovered in 1926. Pursuing his argument, somewhat repetitively, Freud shows us how a traumatic memory can cause displeasure at each cathexis of the engram, but less and less until it is nothing more than a signal. We can see what a well-developed and mature ego can overcome by its elaborative qualities. I won't repeat its description, when Freud puts it so eloquently: *painful* experience generating *displeasure* and *trauma*[1]. Could Freud allow displeasure and trauma an elaborative defence which he habitually refused to pain, although this passage likens them?

We have seen that he refers explicitly in all the texts I have quoted to the difficulty of alleviating or controlling pain and, through his "surprising but essential hypothesis" to its potential ability to self-reproduce and self-aggravate. Freud's position here can be understood from what we know of the suffering he experienced but cannot be fully explained by it. It is too reasoned and consistent. It would be extended in his ideas on the subject of trauma, at times optimistic, when trauma becomes a factor favouring a cure (1937*b*): "There is no doubt that the aetiology of trauma offers the most favourable opportunity for analysis" – and at times pessimistic, when trauma leaves a wound in the ego, "a wound that will never heal but will grow with time" (1927 *Fetishism*).

Algologists will not be surprised faced as they are every day with apparently inexplicable worsening or emergence of

---

[1] My italics

pain. There is no doubt that massive countercathexis of the invasion by pain can mobilise a memory of former pains and narcissistically fabricate a state of cathected suffering with a greater tendency to grow than to diminish. This is the whole problem of psychogenesis and the psyche resorting in some cases to endogenous fabrication of pain, with a paradox, as we shall see later: resorting to pain can have a protective function for the psyche with, naturally, a price to pay.

In brief, here again are Freud's two positions:

- Firstly, displeasure can be improved by means of its memories and even become a protective sentinel for the psyche;
- Secondly, pain has the ability to self-maintain, self-aggravate and even be incurable.

Thus in "Repression" in 1915 it is described as a proto-instinct which brings no pleasure in its resolution other than its cessation and only yields to "removal by some toxic agent or *the influence of mental distraction*". This short, seemingly unimportant phrase which I have italicised is picked up in detail in *Inhibition, Symptom and Anxiety* (p. 101):

> "Also, the remarkable fact that when the mind is *distracted by an interest of a different kind* the physical pains do not occur, even when extremely intense, is explained by the *concentration* of the cathexis on the psychic representation of the painful part of the body."

Distraction or diversion is therefore possible. This is restated in *Civilisation and its Discontents*, which discusses the possibility of decathexis of pain and recathexis of the psyche to another object. What Freud calls concentration of the cathexis may just be this violent "anti" cathexis "of the pleasure principle", the defensive protagonist of the trial of strength which, if we believe his writings, is magnified during a painful experience. The narcissistic libidinal overtension of J. Cournut could then be eased. To decathect and recathect elsewhere is the least that can be offered to a patient in psychotherapy. We shall see the importance of this point in the treatment of patients in chronic pain.

Civilisation and its Discontents shows us a disillusioned Freud sadly reviewing the means available to human beings to battle against the burdens of life, our sorrows and misery – in short our pain:

> "We cannot do without sedatives. We have to have crutches (*Hilfskonstruktionen*)," (Freud, 1929)

He envisages three types: "strong distractions", substitute satisfactions and the use of narcotics. None is good. These are moving pages. We sense nostalgia for cocaine, the chemical way and intoxication, the "breaker of care" that enables one "at any time to escape the burden of reality and take refuge in one's own world ..."

As for the other techniques, they all prove disappointing. Freud mentions yoga, sublimation, intellectual work, art and aesthetics, love, religion ... nothing really works. Little remains except submission. But the man who invented psychoanalysis makes no reference to it to deal with suffering; perhaps, as J.-B. Pontalis says (1988), he considered it too "corrosive"? This would be really surprising and one of the aims of this book is to prove the opposite.

PLEASURE/DISPLEASURE

The workings of the Freudian system are governed by the pleasure principle, which it would be better to call the displeasure/pleasure principle, according to J.-B. Pontalis.

> "We know that there exists in the psyche a certain tendency to avoid displeasure." (Freud, 1895*a*)

But note in a letter to Martha as early as 1883:

> "We try harder to avoid suffering than to seek pleasure."

The context of the second quotation is strange. Freud explains that if we do not fall in love every month or make new friends, it is for fear of the pain we would suffer in separating, losing the friendship or experiencing the misfortune that strikes a friend. Pleasure, displeasure, suffering: we can see the place of these affects in his thought as it took shape.

The problem is that of stimulus and discharge. Freud postulates that stimulus is a displeasure and discharge, by returning the tension to the lowest and most constant level, represents pleasure. Labels such as "constancy principle", "nirvana" and "inertia" show his emphasis on the idea. The pleasure/displeasure principle involves fluctuation between stimulus and discharge. Freud invented protective systems such as the stimulus barrier and attributed defensive functions to the psyche (such as repression) and the possibility of resolution of excessive tension by elaboration. He said that the paradigm of pleasure is the state of the foetus in the womb, sheltered – in theory - from sources of powerful stimulus and displeasure, the act of birth.

This principle is heuristic and Green, for instance, is amazed that it was not invented earlier. It is simple, effective and able to operate the system effectively. However, we shall see that it needed to be modified as it developed, because it raised some questions. Why would the increase in tension always trigger displeasure? Could there not be a qualitative as well as a quantitative aspect? In letter 52 to Fliess, Freud acknowledges that sexual incidents do not all cause displeasure, most are pleasant. This phrase resembles a discovery and is surprising from the pen of a man who had introduced sexuality into psychology. What then of the stimulus due to pain?

> "It has been asserted that all pain contains within it the possibility of a sensation of pleasure." (Freud, 1905)

And in *Instincts* (1915*b*) he accepts that

> "Sensations of pain [...] overflow onto the area of sexual stimulus and induce a state of pleasure; this is why the displeasure of pain can be accepted."

Thus the increase in stimulus, even sexual or painful, can induce pleasure. But having opted for pleasure/displeasure rather than satisfaction/suffering, Freud eliminated pain from his system but not from his thought. Pain followed a hidden trail, sometimes re-emerging unexpectedly, and from this we can discern trains of thought. It would become a parasite of the theory like a fly on a pig until finally combining with it in three articles contemporary with what J. Laplanche called "the 1920 turning point".

Returning to the infant and assuming that life in the womb is a paradise with the tension level at its lowest, we can say that pleasure, in the Freudian sense, is primal. Man's desire after birth is to regain this lost paradise, "assailed by the harsh reality to be faced", as Rimbaud said. This paradise is thus a psychic state which does not recognise reality. Sleep, the baby bird in the egg and the infant, "provided the mother's care is added", come close to this state (*Findings, Ideas, Problems*, p. 137). But this state would not be viable for long. In truth, the three examples are not comparable: sleep is not eternal, the bird eventually emerges from its shell and the infant is separated from reality by the care of its mother. This gives the infant a developed reality with dual valence: both protective - from external reality and of internal needs (especially bodily needs), and also stimulating and creating what I earlier called psychization and humanisation, the two being linked. These two functions, the mother's function as stimulus barrier and her function as the transmitter of psychic life after being the transmitter of life itself, cannot be separated. The stimulus barrier is not a shield, apart from an inherent ability to tolerate a rise in tension levels.

AT THE BEGINNING, DISTRESS

> "You may perhaps be curious to know how one can arrive at the idea that it is the act of birth which represents the source and prototype of the affective state characterised by anxiety." (Freud, 1916)

Freud recounts an anecdote, an amusing incident, which led to a student midwife failing her exam. The question was: "What does the presence of meconium in the waters during labour signify?" She answered unhesitatingly: "That the baby is suffering anxiety", which made everyone laugh. But not Freud, who in his "heart of hearts" sided with the examinee and "her commonsense intuition of an important relationship." The first anxiety state, he tells us, is caused by the separation that takes place between mother and baby, always "ripped from the mother's womb" even if it has had a normal birth, unlike Macduff. By talking of meconium and the anxiety associated with its presence, Freud introduces (perhaps without realising it) the idea of a possible very early affective reaction in the foetus (therefore antenatal), which modern scientific work now confirms (Delassus 2000). We must listen to what scientists tell us, but Freud himself indicated that:

> "There is much more continuity between life in the uterus and in infancy than the impressive caesura of the act of birth would have us believe. The psychic maternal object replaces the biological foetal situation for the child." (Freud, 1926)

However, the "continuity" and "impressive caesura" have to be put side by side to demonstrate the violence of the phenomenon of birth and the absolute necessity for the maternal object to generate what will become psychisation and therefore humanisation in the newborn, starting from the *Hilflosigkeit*, the original distressed state. And further on Freud adds:

> "Therefore the biological factor is the cause of the first danger situations and creates the need to be loved which will never leave a human being." (*ibid.*)

These considerations are important because far from conferring a fatally cataclysmic aspect on the primal distress of the newborn, they make it an initial condition which by its very precariousness imposes a powerful demand for external care which has to gratify the child's physical, affective and psychic needs. In other words the need for a maternal stimulus barrier figure, fulfilling the demand for love and promoting exchanges.

We need to consider this distressed state, which could easily be mistaken for the burden which the reality of life imposes on men, like an inevitable fate. We know of Freud's critical attitude towards Otto Rank, who considered this primal distress of birth as a trauma to be abreacted more and more completely over time, a sort of wound that would scar over. Freud saw this original distress, this traumatic state associated with birth, as the paradigm of the reaction to the danger situation. A reaction therefore to be repeated during all future dangers occurring during "the new forms of existence and psychic development" and therefore in a more progressive and dynamic point of view.

He tended to use the terms distress and anxiety rather than pain to describe this state, but he did use pain in the addenda to *Inhibition, Symptom and Anxiety* devoted to "Anxiety, pain and mourning".

> "There is not the slightest doubt as to the existence of anxiety in the infant; but its facial expressions and tearful reactions lead us to assume that it also feels pain. It would appear to combine what will later be separated." (Freud, 1926)

Unusually for Freud, he is not solipsistic in this text and pain is contained in it within the mother-baby relationship; particularly the repeated reassuring experiences which enable the infant to "distinguish temporary absences from permanent loss" and to learn to comfort itself.

Thirty-one years later he returns to what he had highlighted in "Project for a Scientific Psychology" (1895): the role of a mother towards her child when it rediscovers distress. He had rather forgotten it in the interim, no doubt because he had difficulty imagining a maternal figure marred by the slightest fault. He describes her thus in letter 52 to Fliess:

> "That unforgettable prehistoric figure that no-one can equal later."

THE EXPERIENCE OF SATISFACTION

This chapter of "Project for a Scientific Psychology" precedes the one on the experience of suffering. It is no coincidence that in both cases Freud uses the word experience, which, as the dictionary confirms, no doubt means in this context an operation by which the qualities and value of a thing are judged. Satisfaction and pain are therefore the result of an experience or experiment rather than raw data. The play between the two is the basis for the formation "of a certain state of ø", residual to some degree, of experience of the states of suffering and satisfaction. Freud explains that these are his first ideas about the Ego. The oldest Freudian dialectic is therefore based not on the pleasure/displeasure principle but on the experiences of suffering and satisfaction. Its dialectic of alternations seems relevant to an understanding of the movements of the psyche in relation to its origin.

What happens in this experience of satisfaction? Freud starts from the need for discharge of a stimulus or thrust which tends to be produced by means of the motor function. The internal modification (emotive manifestations, cries, muscular innervations) is ineffective. It is necessary for a "certain external modification (for example supply of food, proximity of the sexual object)" to occur. This is a "specific action" which the human newborn is incapable of performing. This specific action can only be produced "with external help and when the attention of a person in the picture is focussed on the condition of the baby". This generates "a secondary function of extreme importance: that of *mutual understanding*. The original human helplessness then becomes *the primary source of all the moral imperatives.*"[1]

[1] The italics are in the original text.

This mutual understanding is sealed by an encounter. That of the initially uncoordinated gestures of the infant wanting a front view of the mother's breast in order to reach it and the complicit movement of a loving mother who helps to accomplish the encounter. Freud imagines that the sensory stimulus of the baby's skin and muscles produce in the repetition of the experience what he calls a motor or kinaesthetic image, the core of the memory of the affective relationship between mother and child. A mouth seeks a breast; a hand and a gesture guide and accompany it. The baby is unaware but it will remember it.

The "person in the picture", later called the "helpful person" (what a felicitous way to describe the mother!) is what certain patients must have lacked. It is also what they cannot find (because in this case to find would be to rediscover) in the person of the doctor, who cannot be either in the picture about their disorder or helpful. The need to complain is then more important than recovery. The patient does not want to recover and cannot recover. He merely wants to express his chronic state of dissatisfaction.

To some degree dissatisfaction which is prolonged or repeated can be considered synonymous with suffering. It is then easier to understand what Freud meant to say in the chapter in which he showed that the defence against suffering paradoxically self-aggravated it. Pain and solitude unite. The outside help of the person in the picture is needed to relieve the suffering.

The two chapters of "Project for a Scientific Psychology" headed "Experience of satisfaction" and "Experience of suffering" could have given birth to a principle of functioning of the psyche.

Although the pleasure/displeasure principle is theoretically effective, the satisfaction/suffering principle goes to the heart of human affective experience. It produces a memory. Freud says:

> "The traces left by the two experiences undergone ... those generating satisfaction and causing displeasure,

> are the affects and states of desire. These two states are extremely important because they leave motivating forces behind them. [...] Any state of desire creates an attraction to the object desired and its mnestic image and any unpleasant event generates repulsion, a tendency which is contrary to the cathexis of the hostile mnestic image. We have here an attraction and a primal defence." (Freud 1895*a*).

In terms of the defence, Freud introduces an element which can easily pass unnoticed and yet is of very great interest. He wonders how a hostile mnestic image can quickly lose its cathexis and thus be repressed. He presents the idea of another object coming to replace the "enemy" object. A little further on he adds that a "lateral" cathexis can act by changing the course of the current during unpleasant experiences. The idea is that of anti-cathexis allowing repression. We shall again meet this concept of resorting to a related or connected representation to combat the one containing too much stimulus in the excessively clear, the *Überdeutlich*, which is coloured with an intensity borrowed from the representation that one wants to remove. But it is relatively neutral in itself, like the yellow colour of the prairie flowers of Freud's screen memory. That is a diversion and we shall see its importance in the treatment of pain.

To return to the satisfaction/suffering combination. We can see that in this concept the system is no longer binary: stimulus and discharge; it is ternary. There exists a residue of experiences, a memory of the attraction or the repression tendency. Freud calls it a "certain state of ø". This agency impedes discharge and is called the "Ego", he adds.

The ego described here by Freud is capable of cathecting, remembering and so desiring it. Therefore it can impede discharge where the pleasure principle aims at total liquidation of the stimulus, because we need to understand that in this latter system the instinct and desire will disrupt a psyche that aspires to nirvana. We shall see later the difficulty that Freud had in 1924 in incorporating the death instinct and masochism into the pleasure principle.

This is a rather early ego, possibly reaching his work before its time, but it is the result of skilful intuition. It assumes a memory of the cathexes and affects perceived, one of which, we must remember, is suffering, and above all introduces the idea of desire. Affects and states of desire imply "an increase in quantitative tension in ø", which in the other principle is the definition of displeasure. So desire is a pleasure of the ego. But with this we are not in the same world or the same system of thought. The instinct, which renews itself constantly, aims for total discharge. The nirvana of the instinct is at level 0 of the stimulus, says Laplanche (1986). That of the ego is a homeostasis able to accept or even desire discharges and stimuli of greater or lesser importance; these are the "motivating forces".

Above all, the ego is capable not only of bearing the tension but also of retaining it and therefore of dealing with and exploiting it. This retention capability is attributed to masochism later on, in the Twenties. In 1895 Freud's ideas were very close to those which would create the second topic, although it was perhaps more urgent to establish and define the first one. He would not be preoccupied with pain for another twenty years or so. He dismissed it from his mind and his theory, although we have seen that it was stubborn enough to make a few reappearances. At this period he does not anticipate that it can be desired, much less enjoyed, but this does not prevent him writing in a work such as "Instincts and their Vicissitudes" that it could be eroticised like any other sensation and induce a state of pleasure.

I have always been moved by the lines in *The Economic Problem of Masochism* in which Freud anxiously queries his pleasure principle:

> "If pain and displeasure can be ends in themselves and not just warning signs, the pleasure principle is paralysed and the protector of our psychic life is as if under the influence of a drug." (Freud, 1924)

He then introduces an innate sado-masochism coming from the death instinct at work in the organism, part of which is moved outward – sadism – while part remains within – erogenous masochism. This innate masochism becomes "a component of the libido, and yet always keeps as its object the actual being of the individual".

"LOVE IS THE SICKNESS OF THE LAND"

In a pessimistic train of thought, pain is an incurable sickness for Freud, the scourge of humanity by its incurability. It also interferes with his theory and is removed from it. This aspect appears in "Repression", *Mourning and Melancholia, Beyond the Pleasure Principle* and *Civilisation and its Discontents.*

But in another stream of ideas it drives a compelling imperative for processing by the psyche by its resemblance to the instinct. In "Project for a Scientific Psychology", "Instincts and their Vicissitudes", "A child is being beaten" and the 1924 article on "Masochism" it acquires several functions. It participates in the formation of the link with the mother, the repatriation of the instinct towards the ego and the creation of the object and the fantasy. The concept of masochism and the death instinct in particular completely revises the theory, making it more structural. One can understand, as B. Rosenberg did (1991), that masochism can also be the protector of life through its power to bind destructiveness. But I believe that the fact of having dismissed pain from 1895 to 1919, the date of "A child is being beaten", enabled Freud to perfect his first topic and introduce narcissism thanks to an original masochism sensed but not yet formed into a theory.

The last quotation above on original masochism as a "component of the libido" shows the adversary we have to deal with when we treat patients in chronic pain. It denotes the pessimistic aspect of Freud's thought and his nostalgic and masochistic concept of man. The two valences of the "certain state of ø" - ancestor of the ego, the one drawn towards satisfaction and the other towards the suffering it imagines - are the daughters of the *caesura* of the expulsion from Eden and the *continuity* of the earthly paradise.

Both are connected with the maternal dimension. The mother is the origin of both experiences or "experiments". She provides satisfaction and alleviates or removes suffering. This is what the child expects from her and from the unconditional goodness which Freud attributes to her, incapable of imagining her as bad. It is what patients in pain expect of the doctor. The regression which hits them leads them to rediscover the expectation and the appeal which every human being has experienced in the distress of infancy to: "the ancient native land of the child, the place where everyone once first sojourned", says Freud (1919). "Love is the sickness of the land".

Part 2

Clinical Pain

Chapter 4

THE HYSTERICAL TYPE AND HIS SECRET

> *" ... and thus to follow the path that I myself have travelled"*
> *Freud*, Studies on Hysteria, *Preface to the second edition*

THE AMERICAN DRUG DEALER

At a conference on pain, a neurological researcher told the following story:

> An American heroin dealer, himself an addict, decided to escape from the vicious circle of drugs and traffickers. This was very hard to do because of the powerful influence of the drug and intense pressure from his suppliers. He made a plan to leave the city on the Atlantic coast where he lived and go abroad. He gave up using drugs. A few days before he left he had a serious fall on the steep, precipitous steps leading down to a subway station and sprained his ankle badly. He was still under the influence of heroin and felt no pain. He left the United States and began a

long trip around the world that took three years. He met a woman with whom he had two children and later returned to his own country via the west coast and finally went back to his home city. He had been forgotten. One day at the subway entrance where he had fallen, he recognised the exact location of his fall.

- "And immediately experienced ... guess what?" the presenter asked the audience.
- "Pain in his ankle!" the audience replied.
- "No! The classic signs of heroin withdrawal", said the researcher.

And he began commenting on the phenomenon, using chemical mediators as the explanation for the memory of the pain. I remarked that what had been memorised was not pain because there had been none at the time of the sprain or of the withdrawal symptoms and what had happened resembled the "reminiscences" of hysterics, which involved intense participation of the psyche. We know nothing about the young American's psyche, but this short story should make us think. I have told it to show the power that the reminiscent psyche has, with or without chemical mediators, to relieve itself in hallucinatory and motor functions, by giving the affect a means of hysterical discharge.

In this example the process at issue involves an external perception, the view of the staircase. This perception reawakens the inner traces of the accident, its memory. But the accident was contemporary with a particular period in the young man's life which was still vivid due to the heroin withdrawal and the need to escape the dangerous world of drugs, - a turmoil of affects - not to mention the affects associated with the decision to flee in search of adventure due to the decision. The recognition of the stairs forms the second period of the trauma, although it was not traumatic in itself, as with the famous case of Emma. The violent discharge of the affects occurred physiologically, in the complex form of a detoxification syndrome. This is certainly quite amazing and requires total dequalification of the latent affects which cannot be recognised in this syndrome. Therefore it is not symbolic in the narrow sense of the word but is strongly linked to the psychic reality. It is a pain syndrome that is both mental and physical. It consists of anxiety, anguish, various psychic disorders and extremely unpleasant physical manifestations, particularly severe myalgia, trembling, muscle spasms and piloerection.

There is no justification for calling the transition to the physical act of the young American hysterical. That is not what matters. In his case it can be assumed that a debt of violent affects had built up and these had been repressed, avoided and distanced by his flight But the debt was still there and had a date with the ex dealer. The sprained ankle may have been due to a faulty act, but it enabled an "excess" of affects to be both put aside and kept latent, with the complicity of the body. The vision on the stairs after his return – a vision of what, incidentally, because for anyone else there would have been nothing to see - it was the body that was the main seat of the explosion of affects and pain represented by the withdrawal syndrome. The young American perhaps did not have a conversion. I have only quoted this example to show the complicity that can develop between psyche, affects, sensations and physical reactions and the possible interplay of reciprocal collusion and defence mechanisms that can arise between all these agencies – the interplay of their memorisation, their after-shocks and their transformation into something different. Throwing a little light on conversion?

I do not propose considering hysteria further here. It was included to provide a deeper understanding of the (to my mind) inexplicable phenomenon of the psychogenesis of physical pain and its creation by the mind.

SOMATIC CONVERSION AND COMPLIANCE

Mysterious or secret?

Freud guessed that the hysteric protected a secret. He wanted to penetrate this secret and translate or interpret it. He invented psychoanalysis thanks to hysterics and for them: the intrapsychic conflict, the unconscious, the sexual, the trauma, the defence. He constructed the edifice of neurosis. He wanted to see in hysterics the secret of a love story.

This was in 1895, and the secret remains in our time. Freud was right: pseudo proton, primal deception ... Some intuition led him to understand that the hysteric lied and deceived himself and enabled him to discover a truth; that of a psychic reference organisation, a model for the workings of the human mind and the neurosis rooted in sexuality.

A love story then? This is the question posed by J. Lubtchansky (*French Journal of Psychoanalysis*, 1973, No. 3). He was one of the first to question clinical medicine in a different way and to understand the problem of hysterics in greater depth, although Freud, as ever, grasped another dimension behind the flaunted sexual element of his patients. And, writes J. Lubtchansky, he tells us so with Breuer in the message of *Studies on Hysteria*. The affect associated with the causal traumatic event may be rooted in:

- Unexpressed anger;
- Unavenged insult;
- *Pain* due to mourning for a beloved person thought irreplaceable;
- And finally, affects associated with genital stimuli.

I have highlighted the word pain, as I ought also to highlight the other affects, anger, insult and whatever the hysteric offers us that shows (signifier-signified?) that this is not simply a story of love or death but a drama. And that the patients' crude "sexual" element has sometimes been plastered, as if with a trowel, over early and deep narcissistic wounds. On rereading *Studies on Hysteria*, one is struck by the number of deaths, illnesses and other losses recounted by Freud: illness and death of Anna O.'s father; illness and death of the father and two sisters and the many disappointments of Elizabeth V.R., death of the husband of Emmy von N. who was the 13th of 14 siblings, only 4 of whom were still alive, and death of the mother of the children looked after by Emmy von N. These are cases of traumatic distress. They seal the connection which exists between trauma and pain, physical or psychological.

Convert and converse

These related words have deviated from a common origin over time. I cannot imagine that they do not retain some trace of the original meaning. Conversion and conversation are cousins which both derive from the Latin *convertere* (IE root Wer IV), the former directly and the latter indirectly. Hysterical conversion is therefore a language, strong language, body language, preverbal language which seeks to converse:

> "Thus the painful legs also began to "speak" during our analysis sessions." (Freud, 1895*c*, p. 117)

If it is thanks to hysteria that Freud invented neurosis, it is through conversion that he was introduced to pain and became interested in it. By pain in relation to hysterics, I mean both the actual aches and pains and the paralysis, anaesthesia and other physical manifestations which are certainly physical suffering. *Uterus loquitur* said Ferenczi (t. III, p. 64), "the uterus speaks".

Hysterics are not the only ones who use the body to communicate. This is perfectly obvious. Our gestures accompany our words. The stronger the affects, the more violent the gestures. Darwin, quoted by Freud, formulated the principle of "emotional derivation" to explain expressive movements, for example a dog wagging its tail. Freud adds that a patient at the dentist who decides not to move his head "at least taps his feet". The hysteric in crisis therefore makes use of a universal potential (see the case of the American drug dealer).

There are many degrees of conversion. Some appear to be common to people of the same culture. One example is astasia-abasia, the slight muscle movement producing an incipient fall which is so common among hysterics. In this case the somatic compliance is not a pain, it is a sensation experienced at some time during the sufferer's personal life. Perhaps it is a neurological memory of a very distant experience when learning to walk, an anxious imbalance to be overcome and a clumsy movement of the feet appealing to the protective parent or asking to be embraced; a desire to be picked up and carried, the residue of an unknowable experience and the vestiges of an unforgettable close relationship. Conversion is often referred to as an intrasubjective phenomenon which occurs between the psyche and the body with a resolution of the affects and transference into the body. But we must not forget the object. There cannot be conversion without the object. The solitary hysteric does not convert. He wants a witness.

Although acute conversions which only last for a few days or a few weeks are commonly observed, there are also chronic conversions, firmly rooted and sometimes permanent.

Two reminiscences

The hysteric suffers from reminiscences. Reminiscence: "the shadow of a memory" says Robert's dictionary, and Plato: "memory of a previous state when the soul had a direct view of ideas". Fear of a shadow?

We owe the word to Freud:

> "In hysteria, the irreconcilable representation is rendered harmless by the fact that all the stimulus is transferred to the corporal, a process for which I would suggest the name conversion". (Freud, 1894)

This leap from the psychic to somatic innervation – hysterical conversion – is always beyond our comprehension, wrote Freud in *The Man with the Rats* (1907), and he referred to somatic compliance in the Dora case (1905). The two concepts are inseparable. They offer an alliance between the psychic and the somatic which can also be found with the other two categories of psychogenic pain pathology (hypochondria and traumatic neurosis). Each has its specific features, but hysteria seems to offer a model, not so much by the idea of conversion as by that of somatic compliance.

In the article in which Freud suggests the word conversion (*Neurosis, Psychosis and Perversion*, p. 4) to explain critical hysterical manifestations, he pictures the mechanism like this: an event, representation or sensation appears in the patient's ego and evokes such an unpleasant affect that he decides to forget it rather than resolve it, by working through the conflict between the irreconcilable representation and his ego. The ego would even prefer to act as if it had never happened, which makes the process more like denial than repression, closer to forgetting. In brief, the intensity of the affects is such that he cannot forget. The strong representation has to be transformed into a weak representation and to do this the ego must drag the affect away from him. It does this by removing a certain amount of stimulus (the affect). Once separated or dragged away it is converted or transposed into the corporal. But the leap from the psyche to physical innervation does not end just anywhere. It requires compliance from the somatic. How does this compliance happen?

The original German word is stronger than the French translation. *Somatisches Entgegenkommen* means "going to meet, towards", but oddly also "going counter to, going against". The adverb *entgegen* means "against". This linguistic aspect has a resonance which I shall pick up again later, but we can see that beyond compliance the concept is that of an *encounter* between what has to be converted and what receives it into the body. It appears that the reception is not passive and the area of the body is not neutral but is marked by a memory and goes to meet what is coming towards it. There is an encounter of two reminiscences: a representation which the ego wants to ignore and a body which has also been affected at some time. Physical outlet and somatic memory.

How has the body been affected? I can recall some apt quotations from A. Green: "emotional look at the body" and another about the affect: "signifier of the flesh and flesh of the signifier". Certainly the affect is close to the body and the protoaffect which is the raw primal pain and the inevitable starting point for the mother/child relationship is no doubt even closer. So is pain a protoaffect of Return to a time when sensation and affect were combined? This is the heart of our problem. As Freud said, it is the history of the relationship and its successes and its failures that will give birth to the child's psychisation and humanisation.

THE PAINFUL EXPERIENCE OF 'BELLE INDIFFERENCE'

In the conversion phenomenon, the affect is dequalified until it becomes 'belle indifférence'. It loses the unbearability which requires urgent treatment and is transposed and above all transformed into physical suffering, particularly pain in the wider sense. This needs to be preferable to psychological pain. In some pages of *Studies on Hysteria* Freud shares the direction in which his creative thoughts are moving and also the emotion aroused in him by the discovery. He first wonders about the economic gain involved in the process, when discussing the case of Elisabeth von R. in *Studies on Hysteria*. This question had never been asked, but it brought to his mind the idea of pain having a particular function.

The patient suffered from pain in the thigh. Freud explains the reasons for the conversion and its mechanism at length and in detail:

> "instead of the mental pain avoided, physical pains occurred; the transformation was beneficial because the patient escaped from an unbearable mental state, but at the cost of a psychic disorder ... and physical suffering, the pains on which astasia abasia is based." (Freud, 1895c)

A few lines later, as if he cannot believe what he has written, he repeats the question he has just answered:

> "Is it right to focus more closely on the theory and ask: What is the thing that is transformed into physical pain?" (*ibid.*)

And he adds:

> "Cautiously, one can answer: something that could and should have generated mental pain." (*ibid.*)

This is a noticeable hesitation in his thought, which explains the redundancy and above all demonstrates a specific preoccupation with pain. I have chosen this example because mental and physical pain are presented as a sort of alternative or possible choice; as if Elisabeth von R.'s defence – to use Freud's word – preferred the pain in the thigh to the psychological suffering. Physical pain instead of the affect. This is 'la belle indifférence' of the hysteric. The irreconcilable representation has been rendered harmless by the welcoming compliance of a part of the body.

Nevertheless the affect has been dequalified by means of a return, a recourse to the pain of the body. We cannot take this for granted and must perhaps question the logic of pain being accompanied by belle indifférence.

Still on the subject of Elisabeth, Freud tries to understand the reason for the hysterical symptom, its mechanism and how it is determined, in a few pages that bear a resemblance to detective work or archaeology. He repeats his question: Why have pains in the legs replaced mental suffering? The why in the question is more of a how. He says that the neurosis does not create the pain but makes use of an existing somatic pain which it increases and maintains. We know that he liked his concepts to be founded on a physiological or phylogenetic basis, on an origin. He thinks that "a pain with a really organic origin had really existed". The double 'really' is expressive. In Elisabeth's case the pain must have been "originally rheumatic", "perhaps it was a spinal irritation after all", he adds in a note (*Studies on Hysteria,* p. 139).

This prompting of the body to "depsychise" the mental pain by receiving it remains a mystery and does not help us much in our attempt to understand the psychogenesis of physical pain. However, help is at hand at this stage of our thinking. Yes, the conversion silences the thunderous affect, but for the "benefit", so to speak, of another pain – physical – which likewise cannot be treated by mental elaboration. The conversion was necessary precisely because of the incapacity for elaboration and representation of the affect. So it would appear that what was feared was dealing with the affect, probably due to the risk of rediscovering other even more dangerous representations - hated scenes habitually avoided. It was the failure of this avoidance, a gap in the phobic defence, that let in the reminiscence and then the affect - a signal of great danger and trigger of the reflex flight represented by the conversion. Traumatic reminiscence, itself the after-shock of previous traumas.

So there are two movements:

- Firstly, a refusal to make an effort which risks reviving the old relationship with the object and therefore the dreaded affects;
- Secondly, an active, compliant somatic trace which offers itself.

The result is a radical transformation of the affect, which is totally dequalified to the point where a 'belle indifférence' is added to the pain. This indifference is only seen in the long-lasting chronic conversion disorders which shall be discussed later. Whereas the violent "attacks" reveal trance-like states, altered consciousness and dramatisation too impressive not to move, if not the patients themselves, at least the people around them who must pay something back.

TRAUMA AND PAIN

The aetiology of hysteria is directly linked to a real or fantasy sexual trauma and remains traumatic. In 1892 Freud gave a definition of psychic trauma "usable for hysteria":

> "Any impression which the nervous system finds it hard to liquidate by associative mental effort or motor reaction becomes psychic trauma." (Freud, 1892, p. 28)

By adding the idea of invasion of the stimulus barrier which is implicitly contained in this definition, it can be preserved and used to define trauma in general. Note that this definition is also the one for pain in *Beyond the Pleasure Principle* (1920) and does not necessarily involve sexuality, although Freud only spoke of actual sexual traumas in his commentaries. We know that he rejected his theory in 1896. The young women had lied or were fantasising and the adults, men and even fathers were not depraved abusers. Can we be so sure? It quite often happens that female patients mention episodes of abuse suffered in childhood: slight or serious touching, forced oral sex or even penetration. The reports in the newspapers are enough to convince us. Not all these patients are hysterics; some of them have spontaneously integrated the traumas they have suffered into their lives. It obviously depends on the conditions and the violence suffered and the significance they acquire through the subject's traumatic after-shocks. At one time I had occasion to treat young rape victims (The "tournantes" of the time who were raped by gangs of young men in turn) and even in these terrible cases the majority overcame the experience through the psychotherapy they wanted to undergo.

It is clear that hysterics have a tendency to over-cathect memories of sexual abuse (or even to invent them, as Freud thought) and this is actually a trait of their personality. Why?

Having said that, it is not appropriate to classify traumas as sexual or non-sexual. Freud himself, who described three different categories of sexual trauma among 18 cases (*Neurosis, Psychosis and Perversion*), had "indicated as a condition of the pathogenic efficiency of an experience that it should necessarily appear unbearable to the ego and induce defensive efforts" (1905).

What is the hysteric's trauma?

About fifteen years ago there was a great debate within the Paris Psychoanalysis Society (SPP) about depression in the hysteric. A. Jeanneau, the author of a fine report on the subject, postulated that there was no hysteria without depression. M. Fain, representing a theoretical position, maintained the opposite: successful early hysterical identification guarantees that the psyche functions in a way which protects the subject from depression. I am not participating in this old debate, except to say two things.

It is not clear that hysterics, despite their name, have succeeded in their hysterical identifications. We find at the clinic that they are engaged in a constant struggle against a depressive position, with some success. Although it is true that the establishment of a well-developed neurotic state is quite an effective protection against depression, it still remains a part of the human condition. Hysteria enabled neurosis to be described and is its model, but it is far from being the case that all hysterics are neurotic or suffer from neuroses. J. Bergeret has always insisted that a symptom cannot be the basis of a structure and that in *Studies on Hysteria* Freud described a sound theory (neurosis) with the wrong models (patients with symptoms closer to borderline personality or narcissistic disorders).

I do believe that hysterics can be depressed but I think that they are mainly held prisoner throughout their lives in an impossible mourning for archaic parental imagoes and then Oedipus objects. I recall what my friend F. Lévy said during our conversations on hysteria. He wrote (*Crossfire* 1988):

> "We should be particularly grateful to A. Jeanneau for having said that sexuality is hated by the hysteric, doubtless because it necessitates mourning for parental objects."

We must now look into the problem of hysteria to try to understand why and how it may have regressive recourse to the body, and its pain, which touches on difficulties in the early relationship with the mother.

The idea that somatic compliance is an engram with the potential to arouse pain naturally poses the question of the origin of the engram. My clinical experience has long made me think, in line with the work of J. Lubtchansky (1973), that it speaks to us of the archaic misery of hysteria (1974). Others have thought so too, particularly F. Brette (1982, 1985, 1986, 2000), who was very interested in hysteria and trauma. Based on convincing clinical cases, she was able to show how the visible trauma which the loss of an object reactivated in her patients as an after-shock and the lack of mourning for the Oedipus (and parent) figures were linked and constituted the unhappiness of the hysteric. This raises the question of the quality of the link with the primary object and the Oedipus figures. She again explains hysteria in terms of trauma but with loss as the keynote, and repeats a powerful sentence by Freud:

> "Loss of love plays a part in hysteria as a condition determining anxiety, the same role as the threat of castration in phobias." (Freud, 1926)

In some cases becoming hysterical is the best thing to do. "Trauma ... and hysteria to recover from it", she wrote. She showed how analysis could transform hysteria as a disorder into "hysteria as a good thing".

> "It was a case of transforming a lesion that could not be liquidated into sexual stimulus virtually capable of discharge." (Brette, 2000, p. 102)

In an article written in 1974 (*New Journal of Psychoanalysis*, No. 10) – with a title worth noting, "The resentment of the hysteric" – Masud Khan discusses the problem of the nature of the trauma suffered by the hysteric. According to him, if there has been a real trauma in the patient's history, it is not sexual in nature. During the first years of childhood, the hysteric responds to the failings of "good-enough mothering" by precocious sexual development. The child treats this trauma itself by "sexual exploitation of the experiences of the physical ego". A dissociation develops between sexual experience and creative use of the capabilities of the ego, a kind of split.

> "The memories of infancy retained by the hysteric are mainly somatic. [...] In adult life, if the hysteric responds to anxiety by sexualisation, he uses (in object relationships) the sexual mechanisms of the physical ego instead of the affective relationship mode and the functions of the ego." (Khan, 1974)

This sexual solution can only be pseudo-genital and inappropriate. The total lack of understanding between mother and child, the cause of the resentment, is relived paradoxically by the hysteric. The needs of her physical ego have been satisfied and sexualised but not those of her affective ego. Her perpetual quest for sex conceals a childlike, primal demand for love and protection. The logical male response, to proposition her, is seen as a betrayal.

"I needed to be loved and what I got was to be treated like a whore!" said a patient to M. Khan. "The hysteric's basic fear is of psychic surrender to the object. [...] Her inner life is a graveyard of rejection."

Graveyard of rejection no doubt, but also a breeding ground for possible reminiscences. Never give oneself and always reject. Hysterics are on their guard. They remember by repetition and return incessantly to the primal object against whom they had to defend themselves. Their bodies were a blank page to the mother. The physical closeness between mother and child did not produce the mutual understanding mentioned by Freud. Their interaction did not create the necessary symmetry. The repeated physical stimuli had no resonance for the ego other than paraded defensive *pseudo* sexualisation, unusable.

If the sexual element is stimulating (remember that for a long time it was a displeasure for Freud), the response of the hysteric must have intensified the stimuli instead of discharging them. Anxieties have been created, bearing witness to the pain involved in the relationship. To my mind, this is a model for the psychogenesis of pain despite the different mechanism involved in traumatic neuroses and hypochondria. A trace, an algogenic zone has been created and can potentially be reactivated. An algogenic zone, and therefore erogenous and also hysterogenous. A word that Freud never used.

At this point I want to introduce a conceptualisation by Max Schur, Freud's doctor and biographer, which I feel is little known. He assumes a parallel and interdependent development between maturation of the motor system, the development of the nervous system and stabilisation of the homeostatic processes. He says that the result is increasing desomatisation of the reactions to certain stimuli. This produces a tendency to replace action by thought and to reduce vegetative discharge phenomena, the result being control of the stimuli. (Schur, p. 322). He adds that resomatisation of the responses may occur in some regressive states.

I think that the hysteric has not really desomatised and has retained a strong ability to resomatise, not as understood by psychosomaticians who assume the appearance of a lesion, but in the sense of expressive physical faculties. In other words through exaggerated or unusual mobility, neurovegetative discharge (flushing, pallor, vomiting etc.) and sensitivity (pain or anaesthesia).

> I remember a young girl who was brought to me for violent "nervous attacks". Her mother came with a neighbour who I agreed could be present at the mother's request after the end of the first conversation. She told me: "When my daughter does not get what she wants, she cries and has an attack". The neighbour said: "When her mother is not there, everything is fine. As soon as she arrives the child starts screaming".

It is true that "somatisation", expressing through the body, is the only means by which a baby can communicate. We can understand that Schur's desomatisation goes hand in hand with the development that leads to language. There is only one step from a cry to language, said Freud, but it is a pas de deux which requires mother and child to be joined in "mutual understanding" which is rooted in the soma and trusting physical closeness and is open to word play. This did not happen for the young patient described above, as is the case with the future hysterics who retain a return or expressive recourse to the body throughout their lives when urgently needed. An urgent need to protect themselves but also to talk.

M. Khan has shown us the important features of physical closeness and the interplay that may have taken place between the future hysteric and the mother. To my mind, the mother includes the father, the one represented in the mother's head, in and by his involvement. The minor traumas of our early life create thought, but too many traumas, whether excesses or failings, attack and thwart it and leave traces. Trauma also means repetition. Conversion is the means of "translating" the traumatic traces rooted in the hysteric's physical ego. What determines it may be associated with the particular type of specific traumatic distress and to a body which was touched and cannot forget.

This is not the place to examine what may have happened in the history and prehistory of hysterical patients. It has involved a narcissistic identity problem. The primal scene has been harrowing rather than structuring. The picture is made worse by the Oedipus situation caused by an identity in doubt, the violence of the attachment/hatred towards the parent objects and the psychic overheating that it generates. Sexuality thrown out of gear is not erotic, or more precisely it prevents the search for completeness which is a human prerogative.

The sufferings of the hysteric cannot be denied and it is no answer to call them delusions, quite the reverse. It is true that the hysteric's aim is not so much to convince the object or doctor as to exist hysterically in their presence. I do not recall who it was who said at a conference: "I know nothing about hysteria but I recognise it at once when I see it". To be recognised is what appears to be at stake. Unless non-recognition is a means of repetition which greatly encourages the hysteric's problem, like a fly constantly hitting a window but unable to get in. This image evokes a primal scene from which the hysteric feels excluded, would like to be a part of and clings to: a primal scene which has not played the structuring role of the original fantasies.

In truth, when I look back I cannot confuse the large numbers of patients who have revealed their neuroses on my couch with the even larger numbers that I have met at the hospital. Doubtless the neurotics adapted to the couch over time. Freud went through that, and an opistothonos or serious epileptic fit are sometimes a reminder of former "attacks", such as the one in the famous picture "Dr. Charcot's clinical lesson". It shows a beautiful hysterical woman lying gracefully in the arms of the master and apparently in an "altered state of consciousness", as modern hypnotists call it.

Patients like this were described in the *Studies on Hysteria*. They have not disappeared. Freud went to see them *in situ*, in their homes and on their own territory. That is where they can still be found, hospitalised in rheumatology wards for example. They hide their neuroses and express themselves through the body, mainly, in the case of these patients at least, through pain.

I am not sure that hysterics in hospital, whose theatre of expression is the body, and hysterics on the couch who are perhaps more mind based, represent two fundamentally different categories. At any rate they can both teach us something about pain. The patients I have seen in hospital and those who led Freud to write the *Studies on Hysteria* are the same. Hysteria has not aged. We are all strongly tempted to do what Freud did: To try to understand and interpret. The only result is to send hysterics to other shores; to move their suffering elsewhere. I have included a few notes from memory to show that contrary to what people say, hysteria has not changed. It presents its symptomatic excesses and arouses a desire in the other to decode them.

Freud felt the same desire for understanding towards his patients and the same *furor sanandi* for which he later reproached Ferenczi. He never stopped curing pains which never ceased to recur. Put in the same conditions as Freud, faced with the same hysterics and with a demand to give and find a meaning, I went astray. I dislike the term clinical "vignettes", but it illustrates my blunders so well that I am using it.

The beautiful foreigner

This nice young woman with an attractive foreign accent first charmed but then exasperated the doctors in the department where she was hospitalised. They would have liked to diagnose her with sciatica but this did not fit with the approximate, ever-changing course that she described. She was labelled hysterical. The department head wanted to see her with me. She described her problem:

- "It is in my right buttock, the pain goes down the back of my thigh to the hollow behind the knee."

The department head whispered to me: It's a sciatic neuralgia! And asked her where the pain went then ... but the patient interrupted

- "Afterwards it goes three times round my knee, goes back up on the inside, avoids my sex organs, goes up again and grips my left breast."

Disgusted, the department head got up and left. I had to remember that my function in the department was both to help the patients and to enable the doctors to tolerate a certain type of patient. So I stayed, but the patient talked about her country, not her pain. It was there that she had met her husband when he was on holiday. She followed him to France and married him. He worked very hard and she was bored. She often went dancing and enjoyed arousing desire in men:

- I feel their desire when we dance" she told me.

When she then found herself in the bedroom with her conquests, she recovered herself, felt outraged and repulsed them violently. Despite my white smock, she spoke the language of psychoanalysis to the psychoanalyst. She also explained that although she was not very interested in sex, she had been seduced by the Don Juan like appearance of the young tourist who boasted of his many sexual experiences. Her lack of interest in sex did not prevent her imagination being filled with powerful and recurrent images of abductions and even rapes of young women. Two days later she called for me and explained that her pains were not caused by anything she might have told me but by the Lyons climate.

- "Here the sky is grey, but my sky at home is blue."

I said without thinking:

- "Yes, I'm sure your sky is grey!"

She began to cry. The next day when I returned to the department where a whole series of tests had been scheduled, she had left.

- "Due to recovery. She felt cured after seeing you" said the house officer.

She had left a note for me in poor French. She asked me for the address of a psychoanalyst, which I gave her. After all, she had told me what caresses she allowed after three dances and what she did not allow. I could have told her that by avoiding her sex organs and therefore drawing attention to them and by gripping her left breast, the heart side, she was expressing both her guilt and her desire. But it was not important.

Young woman immobile on her chair

She had been paralysed for a month, unable to stand up, and was in pain. Her mother came three times a week to clean, cook and look after the children. Her mother-in-law also came three times on alternate days. She ruled over this little world which she seemed to contemplate from high on her chair, rather haughty and distant. She was the same at the hospital, faraway and impervious to the attention of the doctors. She only confided one thing to me: her mother and her mother-in-law had quarrelled and no longer spoke to one another.

Woman with divided hair

This woman, whose hair was divided into a shaggy part (on the left) and a carefully combed part, held her right hand immobile above her head all the time. No-one had asked her the reason for these two strange habits. I did. She said: "There is something that I have not been able to do for a very long time". "What?" I asked. And to show me what she could not do, that woman who refused to comb her hair on the left, did so!

A man too

He insisted that he was a foreigner, but his strong Lyons accent seemed to contradict this. He told the unlikely story of his life with obvious pleasure. An impressive series of traumas of all kinds. And finally that he had had to marry his grandson's mother! She was a woman who had been abandoned, having had a child by his son and he himself then had a child with her. He delighted in talking about the resultant tortured genealogy and the strangely interwoven generations in which the brother was also the uncle or cousin and the son was his own son's brother. I lost track.

He was suffering from "atypical neuralgia", he was told, sciatica. He did not want to use a stick but was finding it harder and harder to walk. His wife gave him one. "Since using that stick", he said "I walk like a duck". He laughed when he realised that he was also mixing up the genders. When he talked about his bad leg, he called it "the member". The pain he felt came in spasms:

- "The member becomes big, red, swollen, tense and painful. Then comes a series of tremors, the limb deflates and I feel relief!"

The nurses were dumbfounded ...

I have quoted some purely symptomatic illustrations to demonstrate that the descendants of Freud's patients inhabit all the avenues of medicine. These patients often make the doctors smile or laugh. Yet they show the seat of the genuine misery and suffering of hysterics who move us deeply under the mask of indifference. At the beginning of this chapter I wondered whether their facility for painful conversion was prototypical and helped us to understand the mystery of the psychogenesis of physical suffering. The time has come to attempt to answer this question.

THE LESSON OF HYSTERIA

The outlet into the physical mentioned by Freud in the Dora case involves a body that remembers and a representation that cannot or will not participate in the need for effort that the drive imposes on the psyche. No doubt I am not the first to notice that the course of this physical outlet, conversion, takes the opposite path to that of the drive which has a somatic origin and is expressed psychically, via its representations. The representation requiring to be converted "chooses" the return to the body rather than psychic elaboration or a secondary cross repression which would create anxiety, psychological pain or symptoms. The reason for this choice is the mystery of hysteria. In this return we have to distinguish between the point of arrival (the body) the symptom (the pain, or its equivalent, paralysis or anaesthesia) and the feeling: an indifference which is described as 'belle' but could equally be considered paradoxical because it is allied with pain. This contrasts with the painful feelings observed in the other psychalgic disease classifications (hypochondria, post-traumatic pain etc.), as these are usually accompanied by hypercathexis which makes the pain more intense.

The regressive return to the body produces traces which persist and can be reactivated. When I refer to the body, I mean of course the ego body in the sense used by M. Khan (see above). On reading and rereading the *Studies on Hysteria*, one is struck by how Freud touched and felt the bodies of his patients and examined them regularly. He behaved towards them just like a somatic doctor and also administered hypnosis sessions. He had the authority, knowledge, power and activity, which put the patients in a position of obvious or relative passivity. This situation is normal in the doctor/patient relationship, which eliminates embarrassment and modesty, pursued in a climate of confidence that reminds one of the relationship between a mother and a young child. I think that Freud's attitude helped to promote the possibility of conversion and reactivation of very early physical traces that were prehistoric and preverbal.

Freud often gives the impression in the clinical parts of the work that his patients suffered from a current traumatic sexual neurosis because the traumas or series of traumas involved were recent. They were young girls with a difficult traumatic past who were innocent and unprepared for the depravity of adults. He introduced a degree of "constitution". But he wrote in letter 46 in 1896:

> "The scenes leading to hysteria occur in the period of early childhood; before the 4th year, at a time when engrams cannot be translated into verbal images."

Slightly earlier in the same text he says that the residue "intraduced" (as verbal images) does not have psychic consequences but leads to a conversion (*Birth of Psychoanalysis*, p. 145).

WHY PHYSICAL PAIN?

Conversion interests us because it gives us a better understanding of the recourse to physical pain in certain symptomatological organisations. In other words, is the "choice" of physical pain rather than psychological pain "avoided", as Freud says, a speciality of the hysteric? It is hard to imagine an economic gain in this choice, particularly when we recall that in Freud's view the drive and its demand for processing can be psychically liquidated through elaboration, which is not the case with pain.

We must return to the double meaning of the word *Entgegenkommen* (towards and against). In conversion, is it the body which by its compliance summons the representation by going towards it or does it oppose or block psychisation? The compliance is perhaps active and is only asking for an opportunity to profit from the situation and relive and repeat what was traumatic. In this case there has to be an attraction of the representation by the body (the ego body), not just a refusal by the psyche to elaborate. This can only be understood by picturing what the psyche was at the time when archaic traces were instilled. A world of sensations, impressions, frustrated and violent affects, poorly differentiated and therefore poorly symbolised. The concept of "primal symbolic traces" put forward by R. Roussillon (agony, splitting and symbolisation) must no doubt be incorporated here To Freud in the early days, the affect is first close to suffering and then to satisfaction. We must remember the reactions in the form of motor images, of the baby he describes in "Project for a Scientific Psychology". He also refers to "primal symbol as outlet for motor reactions" (quoted by M. Oddy, *French Journal of Psychoanalysis* 1999, No. 5, p. 635). We imagine a primal psyche in which the differentiation between representations and affects was irrelevant, a psyche in an incipient state and therefore close to the body. The return to the body in conversion would then be due not so much to a defensive rejection of psychisation as to a defect, a structural incapacity and narcissistic traumatic traces which are too old and too deep.

Whatever drives these traces to express themselves in a current situation cannot find representations of affects in which to manifest itself other than pain or a physical symptom. We also have to acknowledge that these enable them to hide from a (doubtless dangerous) psychisation, giving the process a protective function in addition to being imperative. The body protects the mind in this case. Can recourse to physical pain be a return to an old and painful experience in which body or psyche had no great meaning? Was there a merging of what would later be separated? This is what Freud says in the 1926 addenda, the most illuminating work that he ever wrote about pain.

Two antagonistic but co-existent phenomena stand out from what I have just written.

On the one hand, a body which a current situation causes to remember old narcissistic traumas through a composite experience of pain; on the other hand, a phobia, a refusal, like a horse at a fence, to face psychic elaboration which risks reviving the old phantoms. By its diversity and the clever way it can behave towards the doctor, hysteria helps to understand the need for painful cathexis of certain subjects, either acutely or chronically.

In all cases of patients in pain, we have to be able to perceive, even if not to understand, the part which only asks to express itself in suffering, as in hypochondriacs or some lumbalgics. But we must forget another part which cannot or will not make the psyche work; although this may involve a refusal, it could also involve a defect, when a child wounded too early has had to retreat into immaturity. Hysteria teaches us the whys and wherefores of a return or recourse to the body, but it indicates a path. Jeanneau says that it "revives the pain to avoid the emptiness" (1985, p. 127). But this possibility can only be hysterical, even if it does not don the cloak of conversion in other psychic forms.

To summarise, hysterical specificity exists. It is the model of neurosis and characterised by conversion. But given that all of us can associate vomiting with mental disgust, as Freud says (*Studies on Hysteria*, p. 2) or neuralgia with some psychic suffering, we can all be represented by the body thanks to "this sort of symbolisation". It is because the body accompanies and represents the mind that it can be a recourse by providing an area of discharge which relieves or clears it.

Conversion is then the point of the demand for consolation. Astasia abasia is seen as a mute appeal and expression of the plea: "Take me in your arms!" ; transmission of the psychic overload to the other with a return to the original innocence.

All pain is regressive; all pain is traumatic. Because of this it can reawaken old traumas, just as an old trauma can find resurgence in pain and express an anachronistic suffering. But the unconscious is unaware of time. This is why hysteria is heuristic.

Hysteria prefers pain to anxiety. At the precise moment of conversion it eludes psychoanalysis. Freud saw that it offered something symbolic. Perhaps, but it was a mortified, split symbolism which only led to an impasse, which was born and died for the needs of the case and for that reason was unusable.

Starting from the situation of original distress of the infant, Freud says:

> "It seems that we find merged in it what will later be separated." (Freud, 1926, *in addenda*)

He envisages pain in terms of the absence and loss of the object and in relation to the maturing process of the newborn:

> "The transition from physical pain to psychic pain corresponds to the transformation from narcissistic cathexis to object cathexis." (Freud, 1926)

Affect, therefore, instead of physical pain, which is the opposite course to Elisabeth von R.'s hysterical conversion. By taking everything, the body protects the mind.

Somatic compliance may be the memory of a time when psyche and soma, sensation and affect, were almost indistinguishable. Freud sees affects (*Inhibition, Symptom and Anxiety*, 1926) as "reproductions of old events of vital importance, possibly pre-individual" and "general typical, congenital hysterical episodes comparable with attacks of hysterical neurosis which are delayed and acquired individually ..."

But this should not cause us to lose sight of the mechanism of revival of pain (no doubt basic, archaic and very precocious) in which a representation is associated with a physical pain rather than an affect. We are all hysterical to some extent. But the hysteric has not forgotten.

The hysteric indifferent? Yes, by always being there: glued firmly to the origins and the parental scene, incapable of choosing. And heartbroken by this impossible choice.

Chapter 5

FOSSILISED PAIN: HYPOCHONDRIA

"You ask why I have so much rage in my heart"
Gérard de Nerval, "Antéros", Chimera

FELIX'S STORY

Félix was a short, stout man, likeable and chatty. I was a consultant at the hospital to which he had just been admitted. His doctor had described him to me as a hypochondriac who had once been very active, not a troublemaker but someone who made many demands, administratively and socially. Was he becoming paranoid? Despite the name I have given him, he looked very unhappy. Unhappy and yet crafty, even rather sly. He had no real idea of why he was in hospital but seemed reassured by the hospitalisation and his doctor too. I had the impression that I had arrived at a moment of crisis which the doctor was unhappy about.

Félix told me his story without prompting. His discourse was marked by a kind of wavering sense of guilt, giving it a particular tone. It seemed to revolve around a specific point which he would suddenly embark on and immediately move away from as though apologising for raising it. Félix was not too sure who had brought him up. His parents were separated. At the age of seven he had been sent into the country as a shepherd. His mother had only visited him once between the ages of 7 and 14. When he was 14 she took him back, but he was uncontrollable:

- "I was naughty and she used to give me a hiding but she didn't hit me hard enough ... so I didn't care".

He then went to live with his father, who ran a small business and decided to "make something of his son". But he still behaved badly and his father used to beat him and one day broke his arm with an iron bar. Félix fled, became a milkman and set up on his own, but took to serious drinking. In debt, he gave up his business and started work at a factory. He married, had two daughters, stopped drinking and worked so hard that he was able to build a house, of which he was very proud. He presented with the dual aspect of a hyperactive man who always had something to do and a hypochondriac, repeating his complaint.

He told me:

- "I will tell you everything from A to X."

That surprised me. Why A to X rather than Z? I claimed to be called BurlouX because he pronounced the x. That did not get me very far, but his wording, which was to be so repetitive, created a small secret link between us, tenuous but strong. One incident sealed our complicity. In one of our first conversations he compared me with the doctors in the hospital who he thought were poor and unpleasant, whereas I seemed to be "exceptional".

- "Some roses for you", he added, but almost immediately began criticising me.
- "Ouch!" I cried!
- "What?"
- "There was a thorn in your roses."

This was my first interruption, which I regretted at once because of its rather ironic tone and its artificiality outside the established structure. But he would never forget it and this, combined with an idealisation of me which proved protective, initially at least, formed the basis on which our relationship developed.

Are hypochondriacs capable of transference? Freud thought that topical neuroses did not lend themselves to it and also doubted the efficacy of psychoanalysis for these neuroses and for pain in general (see for example what he says in *Civilisation and its Discontents*).

My experience at the time tended to indicate the same. Félix had just quarrelled with the doctor who had hospitalised him, which was perhaps not a good omen. But two things had struck me about hypochondriac patients during my medical practice: their unfailing loyalty if one did not try to thwart them and the quality of their discourse, often poetic even if obstinate. None of this implies a potential for transference, but can anything else be expected from someone who has transferred massively onto an organ and a function? I finally accepted being chosen by Félix, not so much as an object but as a screen onto which he could project his two complaints: one hypochondriac, projected within the body, and the other - also projective - originating from external, basically neutral objects. I had the impression that his only internal object was his bent choledochus (which he called "sholédoque") that made his liver diseased and his bile putrefied. His external objects he divided into "nasty people" such as neighbours, colleagues or mates and "nice people", idealised and untouchable: his mother – a saint -, his wife, his daughters and myself. It was almost childlike. I considered the situation favourable and we embarked on a long adventure which I believe helped me to understand something about hypochondria and the opportunities for development that it offers to the analyst.

Things began simply. I listened to his complaints describing his damaged intestines, his defective functions and the fears he had about his the future. He also talked of his period as an alcoholic when he thought he had made a mess of things and it was his own fault. It is remarkable that by simply listening once a week I was able to satisfy the demands of his hypochondria. He stopped all his usual medical treatments and demands for examinations or tests. This was doubtless because I did nothing to prevent him expressing his lamentations, often very colourfully, and paid interested attention to his elaborate theories. I am sure that was not the only reason. A nosographer might think that the grain of sand of Félix's actual hypochondriac neurosis was contained in the "extreme neurosis" represented by his dependence on external objects and the constant projection of his aggression onto them. I prefer to see in my patient the two faces of very early narcissistic suffering which retained its unity for him. My attentiveness also enabled him to through the second - extreme - aspect which proved in the end to be more capable of mobilisation and favourable to transference than the first. The progress of the case confirms this quotation from Freud which I did not have in mind at the time:

> "I now concede what I could not believe before, that analytical treatment can also *indirectly* have a curative effect on the actual symptoms..."[1](Freud, 1890-1920, p. 81)

Ferenczi had written:

> "Pure hypochondria is incurable; it is only when additional elements indicating a transference neurosis are present that psychotherapy can be tried with any chance of success." (*Complete Works*, t. 3, p. 78)

That is the reason why I chose to talk to this patient. It was heuristic; it could not be summed up by any actual neurosis (the grain of sand, as Freud called it). It was always more or less enriched by the true (or false) pearl of just the neurosis and in any case I thought it was his only chance. (Perhaps that was what Ferenczi meant by "double malformation").

[1] My italics

I have to say that my work was made much easier by Félix's experience with his doctor. The dialogue between hypochondriac and somatician is a dialogue of the deaf. One wants to continue his complaints and explain his theories and the other wants to reassure, inform and heal. A desire versus a duty. They remind us of Ray Bradbury's two heroes (in *The Martian Chronicles*), the Martian and the Earthling, who finally manage to find each other. But the meeting does not take place because the body of one passes through the body of the other. Contact is not possible because the species are incompatible. Hypochondria, which Freud tells us must have a reason, does not want to be compatible. The internal scene which the patient describes, a small anatomical and above all physiological scenario, has a history and a cause, hence the insistence on the physiology. In Félix's case, the supposed anatomical defect – the bent choledochus – affected the integrity of the liver and the quality of the bile. There are similar starting points, enriched by the variety of symptoms, that form the tapestry on which the limitless imagination of these patients will embroider and complexify what I have called a scenario, and above all will export it unchanged into the psyche of the doctor, who obviously cannot reconcile it with any patterns. The visual is then involved. Thus I literally "saw" the internal scenario of Félix and felt invaded by a parasite, as he was himself.

I believe that this mutual colourful vision of the intra-abdominal "scene" and Félix's awareness that it was shared consolidated our understanding. I was not an adversary and could then establish the working as a pair. This is common, initially at least, when treating patients in pain and is easier because they feel that the relationship differs from the one with their previous interlocutors. Félix thought I understood and approved of everything he said, and poured out his troubles. No dreams, no fantasies other than the physical equivalents represented by the descriptions of hepatobiliary digestive episodes and gastric pains in which the dominant theme was guilt for his alcoholism.

Félix continued to project his aggression onto his environment. He had great problems with a neighbour who bred noisy geese and with his colleagues for a reason that had occurred in the past. Félix was not a trade union member and did not go on strike. When strikes broke out he was called "yellow" and a scab. He had experienced some very painful moments of "shame". Many similar incidents had marred his life. Nobody liked him and while he was in hospital no-one had come to see him (he had banned visitors!).

I had been under fire from his incessant verbal barrage for some months when one day he told me a strange story about his hospitalisation. While in hospital for his severe drink problem some years previously, he had seen someone die. The vision was hazy but intense. A nurse had sat with the dying patient until the end. It was his first emotion linked to an associative memory rather than to the reality of life and also the first appearance of the fantasy which is so common among chronic pain sufferers, the fantasy of the dead child. He did not speak of it again for a long time, but what followed demonstrated the importance of this small quiver of emotion. Félix was getting better at that time, when disaster struck.

FERENCZI'S LESSON

In his time, there was no-one to equal Ferenczi on the subject of the distress of infancy and early trauma; even ultra-early, as in the expression *Ururtraumatische mütterliche-kindliche Narbe* ("archetypal traumatic mother-child scar") picked up by P. Sabourin in his postscript to the *Clinical Journal* (Ferenczi 1932, p. 292). We should remember this at a time when we are beginning to talk of prenatal traumas (Bergeret, Candilis-Huismanin, *Distressed States*). When we are treating patients in pain, we should keep in mind Ferenczi's impressive articles on trauma which appear mainly in volume IV of his *Complete Works*. On rereading them one is always struck by the truth of a text that now and then becomes a cry, when it expresses distress:

"Quickly! Quickly! What should I do?" (*ibid.*, p. 107)

"Quickly! Help me! Don't let me die in distress!" (*ibid.*, p. 126)

In particular, Ferenczi, the theorist, described the mechanism so often involved in trauma, that of splitting, in different terms from Freud:

> "One has the very clear impression that abandonment leads to a split in the personality. One part of the personality starts to play the role of the mother or the father with the other part and therefore renders the abandonment void and a non-event, so to speak. What is curious in this game is not only that certain parts of the body such as the hand, fingers, feet, genital organs, head, nose and eye become representations of the whole person and the scene on which all the vicissitudes of the personal tragedy are represented and reconciled, but also that a perception is gained of the processes of what I have called "narcissistic self-splitting" in the psychic sphere itself. This history can be interpreted in two ways: on the one hand it expresses the passive resistance which the patient puts up against attacks from the outside world and on the other hand it represents the splitting of the personality into a sensitive part, abruptly destroyed, and another part which knows everything but feels nothing, in some way." (*ibid.*, p. 106).
>
> "Because it is not poetic licence to compare the neurotic's psyche with a double malformation, or a sort of teratoma one might say: a hidden part of the body harbours fragments of a twin whose development has been inhibited." (*ibid.*, p. 96).

This split between a wounded, sensitive part and an omniscient but impassive part corresponds completely to what happens in hypochondria. The patient shelters a monstrous creature in his body, an "allotrion oxymoron" (that is a good and bad body), as I shall call it later. We might add that this kind of dual personality, the result of an attack, is also an attempt at healing. The part that has become clever tries to come to the aid of the bruised part. We recall the famous dream of the "Clever baby" in which the traumatised infant gives wise advice to its parents and other adults, but can also give itself "the task of bringing help quickly to a mortally wounded child ..."

Ferenczi adds:

> " [...] they become good and helpful. Not all of them push mastery over their own pain as far as this, some remain fixed in self-observation and hypochondria." (*ibid.*)

I now want to define how the trauma of which Ferenczi speaks differs from that defined by Freud. Freud stresses the aspect of non-preparation and surprise that defines trauma. The terror then invades the psyche and the normal defence mechanisms are overstretched. The preventive role of anxiety, the signal in other words, is nullified and the anxiety, which is destined for psychic elaboration, is bypassed by this terrifying invasion. The subject is in a state of acute paralysis. The definition of Freudian trauma can be said to be the inability to elaborate psychically, and conversely, if the psyche – which Freud tells us (1914) "performs exploits to handle the stimuli" – cannot achieve this, there is trauma.

Ferenczi's version is different. His clinical experience brought him into contact with patients who were victims of early trauma and chronic traumatic conditions which prolonged or restored the distressed state, the original *Hilflosigkeit* experienced by every human being at the start of life. The maternal environment in particular, which should promote the child's normal process of maturing, has proved deficient, inadequate or even harmful. This resembles Winnicott's theory: something which should usefully have occurred has been lacking. Is this not what Freud (p. 376) realised when he referred to "the need to attract the attention of a helpful person ... to the infant's needs and distress"?

In addition to her consoling function, the mother must be antalgic.

WHAT DOES THE HYPOCHONDRIAC WANT?

- "Like me! Because I hate you!"
- I like you! Why don't you heal me?
- You will never heal me!"

This is the strongly ambivalent, passionate abuse, full of enjoyment, hurled by the hypochondriac at the other person, the current doctor, the forgotten mother... We can understand the reluctance of the medical establishment generally and the lack of enthusiasm of the majority of doctors about the idea of treating a patient like this. Some are able to put up with them and say they like them. Hypochondria is as old as humanity and is apparently the oldest word in the medical vocabulary.

In hypochondria there is no working through the topographical and the repression which might maintain it but would also enrich it. It is repetition of the same thing, the same anatomical-physiological scene. The variations are few, due more to the manner of expression than to the peculiarities of the mechanism expressed. What matters to the hypochondriac is to continue to convince and to maintain his position. A scene now frozen once existed and survives by repetition. It has forgotten what it witnessed but is to amnesia what insomnia is to the dream. A rejection. An insistent, obdurate and in some respects triumphant rejection.

To convince and triumph involves the need for an interlocutor or even an opponent, and we are then taken to the very heart of the arena where the hypochondriac and his doctor confront each other.

The relationship between the hypochondriac and his doctor is therefore a necessary one. The hypochondriac cannot do without it. He forces it on the doctor. It is a relationship of a particular type which ignores the conventional doctor-patient rapport. This is based on a therapeutic alliance involving mutual understanding sufficient to establish effective cooperation. Doctor and patient are agreed on the objective to be achieved, healing in the best cases, and the therapy to be applied. The natural counterpart to the presumed skill of the doctor and his treatment will be the patient's trust and a certain degree of regression. To receive care is to rediscover the period of maternal care that all humans have experienced. This period may have been charged with pleasant nostalgia and regression is then easy. Equally, it may have been marked very early by the absence of what Freud saw as the basis of the mother-infant relationship and the start of the child's development: the mutual understanding which allows and is allowed by satisfaction. This is what seems to be lacking in the exchanges with a hypochondriac: he does not want to understand; he does not want to be understood. He is eternally unsatisfied.

Basically, the hypochondriac is continually being told by the other person, the doctor, that there is nothing in his hypochondrium, while he maintains that there is something. The confrontation is between two people who know: the man whose job it is to know hypochondria and the patient who knows everything and wants an adversary to match him. Certainty based firmly and paradoxically on profound doubt.

I am not saying that a hypochondriac patient does not experience anxiety. He is constantly casting doubt on the reassurances offered by the doctors, but his apparent nosophobia is founded on a basis of certainty, that of his theory. The hypochondriac is not nosophobic. We often read in the psychoanalytical literature about work on hypochondria when it is really about nosophobics, whose problems are quite different because they try to cathect an unconscious aggression by means of guilt and fear of disease. Hypochondriacs *know* and although they ask to be healed, which is what doctors hear, their main aim is to express their chronic dissatisfaction. They hardly ever consult psychoanalysts and the latter are often reduced to referring to just one moment, a sudden hypochondriac episode in the complex history of their patients, when asked to talk about hypochondria.

If trauma is repetition, then hypochondria is certainly traumatic. The misfortune is that the hypochondriac knows nothing of the cataclysm that once devastated him and yet recounts its effects endlessly. The analyst can try in vain to pick up some traces of a thread that might lead him somewhere from the patient's wordy descriptions of the harm done to him. This raises the question of the language used by the hypochondriac patient. It describes the symptoms, sometimes very vividly, but these symptoms are not symbolic, Freud tells us. What chance is there be of attaining some polysemy of words that might enable an obdurate psyche, deaf and thunderous, to work things through?

I mentioned earlier that there is a visual element in what is expressed by these patients' words. There is so much repetition and careful description that the interlocutor suffering them is forced to visualise the scene depicted to him. The patients' affects are so forceful that one finds oneself frozen at the scene, as the scene is frozen in its repetition. What are the affects? All the authors rightly emphasise the anxiety of hypochondriacs, the anxious wait to speak, like Freud. For my part I prefer to emphasise the feeling of certainty and triumph contained in their words. This underlines their resemblance to victims of both paranoia and melancholia, and also to some degree fetishists.

Therefore hypochondriacs take us into in the narrow relationship framework imposed by them and keep us there. Although there is very little or nothing to be done with the colourful images they display to us, perhaps we can think that the relationship reflects and repeats a previous situation. This situation must also have been marked by violent primal affects which are hard or impossible to define, and their former presence is felt once again, here and now, in our presence and is transmitted to us. The images are present because they were contemporary with these affective states. Violence of affects and violence of images, linked by contemporanity, without the mediation of language forging links between the two kinds of violence or with the rest of the psyche. It is like standing in front of a picture of a battle without being able to hear or read an account of it. This implies that the situation that was traumatic was very early, certainly pre-language. At least this is what I shall try to show.

What doctors do not understand is that their presence is absolutely essential for the hypochondriac to function.

HYPOCHONDRIAC SCENE AND AUTOEROTICISM

The hypochondriac's game with himself is a type of autoeroticism and we have to examine its peculiarities. In *Three Essays on the Theory of Sexuality* Freud describes the mythical moment of the appearance of autoeroticism:

> "At the time when sexual satisfaction was associated with food intake, the drive found its object outside, in the mother's breast. This object was later lost, perhaps at the very moment when the baby was able to see the whole of the person possessing the organ that brought it satisfaction. The drive then becomes auto-erotic." (Freud, 1905*a*)

And later comes the famous phrase:

> "To discover the sexual object is really to rediscover it." (*ibid.*)

The French translation "see the whole of" does not accurately render either the German *bilden*, to form or constitute, or *Bild*, which is the image. The German meaning is closer to the origin of the work of visualising and fantasising associated with the discovery of the whole object, via hallucinatory realisation and introjection. That is to say, closer to work of representation which is simultaneously a loss, that (of the role) of the partial object, and an arrival, that of the object and therefore of the subject himself and access to fantasy.

As J. Cosnier commented (*French Journal of Psychoanalysis* 1977, 5-6, p. 1020), autoeroticism directly releases the sexual drive from its supports but finds itself in a situation of conflict on two levels: "in the guilt towards the parental objects and in the narcissistic lesion which it tries to heal by its fantasised accompaniment". The lesion is linked to the child's dependence and impotence. In this way little Hans shares "in all aspects of parental coitus through his bisexual identification fantasies". This is true in good cases.

What Freud describes is the moment, again mythical, when the object of desire and the object of need separate. This presumes a degree of maturity in the child's psyche. Between the initial autoeroticism, suckling, which is satisfaction on the spot through the baby's own body, and the fantasy accompanying autoeroticism when the object has taken its place within the child's psyche there is a process which requires parental input.

Being with hypochondriacs enables one to picture what has happened between them and their mothers, as we have seen in the clinical illustration above.

We can imagine a situation of distress that leaves the child without recourse:

- neither external, because the mother proves powerless to soothe the distress or even triggers or worsens it;
- nor internal: the child is unable to construct a sufficiently reassuring image of the mother and its other objects.

It cannot relive them when they are not there, either by imagining their presence or playing with its memories and daydreams. Nor can it imagine them negatively in their presence and prefer solitude by going back to its psychic functions. Distress is nothing but a series of violent stimuli that do not receive reassurance. The theoretical concept of stimulus barriers which Freud used is a metaphor and should not be seen as an armour or shield. The stimulus barrier is the power to control and assimilate the "excess" of stimulus by the "normal channels", as Freud said, i.e. the channels of psychic elaboration. The first stimulus barrier is the mother and what is exchanged between her and the baby in reverie, attraction and sharing that promotes this process of psychisation and, all-in-all, humanisation.

This process does not always take place and when this is the case the autoerotic fantasy is poor and repetitive. It cannot be transformed into dreaming and allow the psychic function to take root. The stimulus will only have the body for discharge and two channels are then possible:

- Painful sensory phenomena;
- Or motor phenomena such as hyperactivity.

As we have seen, Félix chose both.

Everything depends on the means of surviving the loss and absence. If the baby has formed a sufficiently reassuring internal image of the mother, it can occupy itself alone when she is not there. If not, without an internal object of recourse and succour there will be a mutual lack of comprehension, anxiety and, worse still, distress. The ability to imagine absence prevents experiencing it as depression/pain or ill health.

In Ph. Jeammet's excellent article "The Enigma of Masochism" (2000), he compares three solutions to compensate for the mother's absence.

- In the first the baby has "sufficient internal resources". It is peaceful, sucks its thumb and "develops an activity of recall of pleasant memories and sensations". "Mental representation", "recall of the mother as such is not necessary". "She is present in the very quality of the pleasure enjoyed by the baby." "Psychic function is a substitute for the actual people around it."
- In the second case, the baby cries. "It is in a situation of dependence". It needs the mother's actual presence so that its psychic function is satisfying and "the good objects prevail over the bad". These children can become temperamental and tyrannical "making their mother dependent on them in turn".
- Third solution: the child "does not have the resources to cry or call out". It replaces the lack of

> recourse, both internal (the autoeroticism) and external, by self-stimulation of its body "(rocking backwards and forwards, hitting its head, tearing its hair ...)

> "The child then develops an activity of seeking sensations which are characterised by being always painful and having a destructive dimension." (Jeammet, 2000)

Ph. Jeammet enables us to focus on a continuous area which has no precise boundaries. We can localise the particular territory of the hypochondriac within that area by trying to understand it within the framework of the relationship with the mother and the family background in general. Quite obviously, the hypochondriac's autoeroticism makes the first solution impossible.

Freud (1914) starts from autoeroticism to "present" narcissism. To illustrate it, he refers to pain "when the soul shrinks to the narrow gap of the molar", physical illness, hypochondria and being in love. Always cautiously biological, he thinks that the hypochondriac must be right and organic manifestations cannot be lacking in his case. He seems quite triumphant when he finds a model "of a painfully sensitive, modified organ...without being diseased in the usual sense: it is the genital organ in a state of arousal". Further on he refers to "a stasis of the libido of the ego". It is hard to imagine the why and how of this stasis. The enigmatic Freudian metaphor seems to be taken too far. Why and how stasis? But it allows Freud to pose a relevant question: "Why should this stasis of the libido in the ego be experienced as displeasing?" and painful. We have to consider this short sentence - which is not often taken up by authors interested in hypochondria - because it is extremely rich. Freud thought at the time that an increase in tension and displeasure were synonymous. But is this the case with sexual tension? And is the aroused sex organ painful? We know that Freud did not come back to these theories until 1924 (but he acknowledged in the letter to Fliess of 6-12-1896 that most sexual encounters were pleasant). The question he poses is the one that interests us: possible painful sensations in a part of the body that is free of lesions. Whether or not there is a change in the organ does not seem to me to be very relevant. Freud always insisted on a biological root. In hypochondriacs it was the "stasis" of the libido and in hysterics he thought that "a pain with a real organic origin had really existed at the beginning". This is also what patients think and they - and Freud - may be right. But what can we do about it?

WHAT CAUSES THE BODY'S SILENCE?

What has happened? We can look at the problem in reverse and ask with M. Fain what causes the body's silence and understand it as he does as "a continuous perception of reassuring impressions". This to me is a beautiful image of the protective and comforting mother. The hypochondriac sensation must then be a failure of this silence and the "response to the perception of a failing at the heart of these reassuring perceptions; a response doubtless aiming to combat the anxiety associated with this perception of a deficit and not succeeding". The clinic confirms this. When the hypochondriac forgets himself, ceases his litany of complaints and starts to talk about something else, it is important to note the kind of small relational incident that will plunge him back into his depression, like a small gold nugget in a torrent.

Freud and Piera Aulagnier use the same image to picture the "mutual understanding" between a mother and her baby resulting from the baby's motor appeal and the mother's response. The image is that of the meeting between the mother's breast and the baby's mouth. Freud imagines that while feeding the baby forms an image which he calls motor or kinaesthetic. Freud speaks of the meeting of two mnestic images. The first is perceptive and is the memory of the traces of the desired object, the mother's breast seen from the front. The second image is motor, or kinaesthetic, which is a better description of the sensory-motor aspect. For example "the memory of an experience felt by chance while feeding, a particular movement of the head which changed the front view to a side view". Due to its recalled experience, the baby can "make the reverse movement to obtain a front view" and grasp the breast. It is important to note that the first image, the visual perception trace, is on the passive side, while the second, through mobility, opens up the area of activity and action in relation to the world to the baby. And we imagine the mother's gesture accompanying or even helping that of the baby and sealing their mutual understanding.

Piera Aulagnier (1975), with her complementary object zone concept, also starts from an "initial experience of breastfeeding which brings a mouth and a breast together". This is a combination of: satisfaction of the need, swallowing of an object taken into oneself, the encounter through sensory object organisation, a source of stimulus and a cause of pleasure (p. 61). She places much greater emphasis than Freud on the affect, particularly violence and destructiveness, that can alternate or co-exist with pleasure. She says that the phenomena of displeasure and suffering are equally present. The "pictogram" is much more explosive than the Freudian images. "The absence or inadequacy of the object due to excess or deficit" will not only render the object bad but also the "zone" in its pictographic record. The scene becomes: "a mouth trying to tear the breast, a breast trying to tear itself from the mouth" with "mutual rejection between zone and object and also between representing and represented agency", which is violence "which is accompanied by the desire to destroy the object and annihilate the erogenous and sensory zone and its activity." This represents a destructive version of the Freudian motor and kinaesthetic image under the aegis of mutual understanding.

What does the scene recounted endlessly by the hypochondriac conceal? I recall a long conversation I was fortunate enough to have with Piera Aulagnier. When I told her that Tausk thought the body was the primal object, she said to me that it was also the primal persecutor and therefore the primal cause of pain. I then moved on to Freud's first ideas of the ego which were based not on the pleasure-displeasure system but on the facilitations (a certain state of ø) created by the test (!) of satisfaction and test of suffering that were their ancestors (see "Project for a Scientific Psychology"). It is true that pain is primal. The primal function of the mother, to give her baby sufficient satisfaction, is to "depersecute" it of its own pain, provide it with continuous comfort, assure and reassure. As we shall see, deficits in this function "are the basis of much of the chronic pain in adulthood", as a paediatrician asserted at a conference (and was heavily criticised). They are also the origin of a certain type of mother-baby relationship which forms the core of hypochondria. What the hypochondriac says reveals the result of the process: a belief in an anatomical imperfection and a functional disorder as evidence of a body that was once attacked. In particular (which the patient takes as proof) a sensory experience which is not just painful and confirms the reality of the harm suffered. As I have said, unlike in hysteria the harm is not symbolic of a psychic event, trauma or affect. But the need to convince, the fervour, the verbal intensity, the careful description and the images used to "show" the tragic scene played out in the body – and I stress the visual – must be the vestiges of an old, unheard violence. We can easily see the polyphony in this frenzy of affirmation of the disease, the deaf ear turned to the other person, the doctor, and the persistent refusal to accept the reality that would bring relief.

We can see that Piera Aulagnier agrees with J. Bergeret and his "fundamental violence". To reiterate, he thought that although fundamental violence, resembling a survival instinct – the Freudian *Bemachtigung* – can be destructive in its effects, it is not in itself destructive and is not a desire to destroy. The function of appeal that it incorporates must be identified in the baby.

Either a motor (and kinaesthetic) image or a pictogram, but certainly an image. Freud placed more emphasis on the image (it is again motor) and Piera Aulagnier on the affect (but she refers to a pictogram, therefore also an image). What happens to this image in the future hypochondriac?

We have to imagine that in the distress of a maternal relationship that lends itself to it, the future hypochondriac baby is gripped by a sensation or perception and has cathected it by embodying it, in the true sense. If the experience of satisfaction causes representation via hallucination, enabling the baby to wait for the object, how can we imagine the traces of distressed states felt and reactivated by the absence, loss or poor quality of the object? We go back to what Freud called "a certain state of ø taught by the experience" (in *The Birth of Psychoanalysis*, p. 340) and modelled by the sequence of hostile or satisfying experiences. The object contains a "non-assimilable part": *das Ding*, the thing, and another revealed to the ego by experience and allowing understanding. We know that Freud tended to invest the mother with every desirable quality, which was no doubt why he disregarded maternal transference in his cures. And yet he wrote as follows after what is quoted above: "In the first place there are objects (perceptions) which cause crying because they cause suffering" (*ibid.* p.372). Freud adds that the association of the cry with the perception is a combination which can increase the hostile nature of the object, and he sees the possible emergence of the first conscious memories associated with their unpleasantness.

The association of the cry and the perception and the related existence of a motor or kinaesthetic image, calling for "specific action" from the unhelpful and failing object awakens thoughts about the psychic traces formed by the experience of distress. If there is continuity between satisfaction, image, representance and representation, fantasy and fantasising, what happens to the image when distress outweighs satisfaction? I quote from C. Chabert:

> "A powerful affect, distress instantly evokes the image, no doubt to contain the excess, the risk of overflow ... and the risk of acute pain." (Chabert, 1999).

In hypochondria this risk has not been avoided and the image is not the fruit of satisfaction, it is a defence against distress. It is like a plant that grows spindly in arid soil for lack of good fertiliser.

This image originates from the body and is part of an archaic situation in which the distinction between representation and affect is not relevant. It is the source of what will become the hypochondriac scene. It occurs in an immature psyche under stress and originates from perceptions that are too violent to be metaphorised in representation. It is an early traumatic situation of over-affect, great pain (or what will later be felt as pain), little or no representation, replaced by an image; this situation describes trauma and Ferenczi's colourful and expressive view on the split seems very heuristic. We can hypothesise that the violence of the situation splits the immature psyche into, on the one hand, a "knowing baby" who will later fabricate theories and knowledge about the organ and, on the other hand, an innocent being that clings in its distress to an image which - it is now important to establish - is sensory and motor and therefore rooted in the body. It is on this split that hypochondria is built. The image will generate the scene and the knowledge the discourse.

HYPOCHONDRIAC THEORISATION IS A SEARCH FOR MEANING

Many children experience early suffering without becoming hypochondriacs. An early trauma can be the preliminary blow with later after-shocks, as we shall see in some cases of traumatic neurosis such as lumbalgics, but the course of hypochondria is quite specific.

The sensory-motor sensation cathected, memorised and turned into a psychic image is of a particular type in the future hypochondriac; it is marked by pain, pain without consolation. The sensation of pain will be rooted chronically and permanently. It has a function of appeal but no longer expects a response. It becomes a precious part of a masochistic narcissism that feeds on its repeated affirmation. The image has already become a translated sensation, an incipient psychisation which presumes a small shift to allow the modest beginnings of self-observation, or rather a *view* of the pain. Does a sensation which can find neither meaning nor satisfaction and which retains its potential for stimulus become pain? A. Beetschen in an excellent article on Hamlet (*New Journal of Psychoanalysis*, No. 39, p. 243) asks this question: "Does the stimulus take the place of an impossible sadness?" I would add 'or of an impossible mourning', which is the case with the hypochondriac.

This psychic construction from the body cannot be understood unless it is again set within the framework of the relationship with the mother, even if this is a failure. F. Perrier said that the hypochondriac "has become his own mother, alienated from the symbolic maternal world to fall pregnant by himself as the phallic child". It is true that pregnancy fantasies are quite common among hypochondriacs. This is due to the failure of the attempts at independence caused by the father's absence. As we saw with Félix, what he missed most was a father. But it is also true that this construction of such a specific internal world retains a maternal valence.

The sensation felt at the beginning was not necessarily associated with the pain of a particular organ. Distress is wholly pain. The organ that becomes painful (the famous libido stasis) becomes the witness to the pain. The witness but not the symbol, even if it is the mark of, or retains an unelaborated trace of, what the relationship between mother and child was like. The "choice" of organ, however random it is, may be the result of excessive maternal care or the opposite, the memory of the child's unheard physical complaints. Hypochondriac symptoms often involve the digestive system and affect what is under the hypchondrium and the ribs, and this may not be coincidental. The first relationship is digestive. Does a young mother not feel anxious that her baby will not "take to" the breast?

I believe that in some cases the mother has also cathected the shared sensation, but in anxiety. Here is an example:

> As a very young general practitioner I often saw a mother, herself a hypochondriac, who had focussed her anxiety on burping her baby. The burps took too long to come or were insufficient or not strong enough, never satisfactory. The mother would manipulate the baby's body (head down, pressure on the stomach) but that did not help; the father laughed in the corner. By chance more than twenty years later when I had become a psychiatrist and psychoanalyst, I met my young patient again, a perfect example of the "worrying well", according to the doctor who had referred her to me.

Whether cathected by the mother or not, the child feels kinaesthetic sensations which certainly belong in the relational space between it and its mother. Some may form a complaint. The fate of the complaint addressed to the mother differs according to whether it is heard or unheard, ignored or comforted. Is a space created in both protagonists for the other? The mother's action may be a seduction in the etymological sense of the word *se ducere* "to mislead". A particular repetitive kinaesthetic sensation may be *chosen, made painful.* It is not transitional or rather does not find the object because it is not there. The game is and remains autoerotic if not masturbatory. Paradoxically, the pain then becomes a self-calming, anti-pain process through its illusory control which develops into a theory.

From the cry to language there is only one step, wrote Freud at the beginning of "Project for a Scientific Psychology". When this step is taken, when the child can put words to its sensation of pain and when the age of childhood sexual theories is reached, an eroticised, overcathected theory is constructed in the enjoyment of their flights of fancy. If the periods of latency and adolescence are silent, then the theory starts from the conquest of the psyche while preserving a part of it. Part for all. This is self-sacrifice.

What has been incorporated is an illusion, a child-mother composite; Incorporative identification of an infanticide part of the mother and her child. It is a monstrous figure combining the archaic oral mother devouring her child and the dead or dying child fixing the scene to keep her and stay alive. We have to picture an anxious mother too inclined to worry, maybe distant and icy, or even a hypochondriac herself. Certainly deaf to the sorrows and appeals of a baby that has only pain by which to express itself and appeal to her for help. The baby has created a teratoma or allotrion oxymoron (good and bad foreign body), a monstrous "other" in himself, at the cost of pain.

This pain is a vestige of the violence of the affects created at the heart of their relationship and the pain unheard by the mother. In this situation the baby has tried to regain control and has swallowed its mother and then faecalised it. What could and should have been the inner object has been replaced by the organ, diseased and painful but still alive, battered and bruised but functioning, between life and death.

In this extreme condensation we are at the limit of opposites which lose their meaning. The mother is destroyed and preserved, the "mortally wounded" child is still alive, activity and passivity are merged, as are love and hate.

It is the terrible encounter between the infanticide mother and the child not deterred from its archaic desire: to kill the love object. In the tomb of the hypochondriac, the eternal vigil over the immortal dead child goes on.

The auto-narcissistic split referred to by Ferenczi has been a desperate salvation, the best possible defence. The damage can be seen. Although less visible, the reality of the salvation can also be estimated. The internal object has been replaced by the diseased organ.

One question arises: Why is a sensation which is initially physiological and repeated chosen, cathected and "made painful". Why does it become a mental image, then a scene, generating a thought then a theory, in a hard and independent facilitation with little or no connection to the network of representations? Could it be the greediness of masochism?

This would explain retention of the accumulated stimulus, an intense masochistic and narcissistic cathexis which has a specific drive purpose. The famous "libido stasis" on or in the organ would then be self-sustaining. This is Ferenczi's split. The trauma has not destroyed the subject, who resembles part of a dead tree which starts to grow again.

What fascinates me about hypochondria is the importance of theorisation for the patient. He clings to his theory even more closely than to his pain. The original petrified fantasy has given birth to an idea which immortalises it. The requirement for fantasy then yields to the need for theoretical abstraction, at least in this part of the split. This is where it is not enough to understand the hypochondriac and his desire not to be cured only as masochism. I quote from J. Cosnier who poses a question rarely asked: When do they want to be healed and when to generate and create?

> "The representation-aim of curing conflicts with the limitlessness desire to generate." (Cosnier, 1987, p. 155)

F. Perrier (1959) noted the self-generating fantasies of a hypochondriac patient (actually psychotic). He said it was impossible to separate this desire for creativity from the painful autoeroticism that these patients exhibit. By being both the patient and the doctor, being active and passive, providing all the polarities of the ambiguous and worrying illusion of early life, the hypochondriac fabricates the mother-baby unity of his origins. Starting from this point, a strange primal scene, he wants to create his mother and give birth to himself and does not distinguish between this movement and a desire for destruction. This is doubtless where the unending aspects come from.

FELIX'S DEPRESSION

Two events occurred:

1. One of his two daughters had to leave the area for work reasons and the other planned to marry and move to the other end of the country;
2. He became registered disabled.

Three of his points of reference and anchorage disappeared. He had known about it for several months but was incapable of anticipating it and experiencing preventive anxiety. He remained indifferent to these events and yet talked about them repeatedly. The important thing is that I was afraid for him and instead of him, counter-transferentially.

He suddenly decompensated with incredible abruptness. I had to reinforce my treatment, increase the number of sessions, recommend medical treatment and be more involved in his problems (administration, papers etc.). During an initial period when he never talked about the new conditions of his life of solitude and idleness nor of his distress or what was causing it, he began losing weight and eventually became very thin. He reserved his hypochondriac aspects for a somatician, materialising his structural split, and showed genuine hatred towards him in a kind of lateral transference. A sort of inverted nosophobia made him want "terminal cancer" and "he" could find nothing wrong with him.

I was faced with a man in the negative. He did nothing, wanted to die and said not a word about his mental suffering. He was just the blank screen of an interrupted film. His obvious depression found no words. As for myself, I could find no effective means of gaining access to his manifest aggression and therefore sense of guilt. We can see the part that physical pain and recourse to the body can play: protection from an unbearable process of working through things psychically.

I explained to him that if he had that cancer it would be incurable and if he died we could no longer see each other. I never imagined when I said this that it would have such a profound and violent effect. Death was a separation. The problem of separation seemed more real to him if he was the one who disappeared. This puzzled him and the fact that his medication was antidepressants (!) finally made him aware of his depression, but in a rather intellectual way. He would introject it through action.

He had replaced his former alcohol dependency with "my" medication (actually prescribed by a psychiatrist). Sometimes he took an overdose and fell into lethargy, but not for long enough for his wife to notice. He called it "mini suicide" and it was our secret. "Oh doctor, if you only knew how good I feel when I do it!" he said. Although his behaviour troubled me greatly, these words touched me. This artificial slumber, this great happiness won over too harsh a reality, reunions with an ideal mother never known, were combined with the trust he had in me and his gratitude for the interest I showed in him. This was the beginning of transference – acted out because it was with "my" medication that he "committed suicide", but real. After that it was between him and me. He began putting on too much weight, became almost obese and gradually resumed his hypochondria, complaints and projections. He could be aware of his own aggression and anxiety. He became hard to tolerate within our relationship.

But he preferred action. He had repainted his garage and made a large red stain on the ground which he could easily have removed with trichloroethylene. He did not, and walked round it jubilantly "I don't give a sh— what anyone thinks" he said, but why?

The episode of the rotivator was more worrying. Félix was literally afraid to start up his rotivator, or more precisely not being able to start it up. He used a product (quick start) which made the operation easier but risked "wrecking" the motor over time. Yet he had no problem with his lawn mower which had exactly the same starting mechanism. So he was using a product that aided starting but was corrosive. The motor gave up the ghost. Félix, feeling very guilty, went to see a mechanic. Consternation! The cause was quite different. Félix, whose job it was to fill machine tools with oil, had not put any in his rotivator! But why this attack by him on the rotivator and why this anxiety, he wondered. Fear of the object, fear in face of the object and a secret desire to attack it, thus his prehistory repeated itself and his relationship with me was explained or at least made clearer. Félix was becoming interpretable. I began making approaches which he accepted.

The rotivator and the mower were gradually sexualised. The mechanism of the former was much more complex and inaccessible than that of the mower, which was much easier to see and dismantle. The rotivator evoked the hidden anatomy and the secret, worrying internal physiology of the female, the invisible functioning of the maternal feminine referred to by A. Gibeault (1995).

I did not follow this trail in detail, considering it more as an indication of Félix's progress along the path of symbolisation and complexification of his psychic apparatus: colleagues who were red, the red stain by the garage were then registered differently. Félix, the Yellow, the Fox, played with yellow bile and the defective physiology of the bile ducts and their anatomy, visual and above all visible in the male genital organs. Yellow bile, red stain and worrying workings of the motor. Félix had less need to project his inner scene outwards and with less anxiety. Could I find an opening that might help him work through things psychically?

Small mental images were generated, based on colours: the yellow of the bile and the yellow of the strike-breaking fox were in conflict with the red of the aggressive trade unionists barricading the factory gate. The elbow (invented by Félix) of the choledocus recalled the elbow fractured by his furious father. The red garage stain acquired a density and soon a new meaning. Precipitated, as Freud said, by the "conditions" of the fetish. Our work became more substantial and Félix developed a taste for it.

He could then attack me much more. My hydrangeas were miserable, my roof boarding was in a bad state, and my string courses were shabby. He criticised me. I was no longer the ideal being of earlier. After the distinction between dangerous feminine and reliable masculine, he discovered that it was possible to be aggressive towards me, but for quite excusable reasons, so that aggression and guilt became part of the psychotherapy "game".

The situation deteriorated due to two incidents.

Firstly, medals were to be awarded to employees with thirty years' service. Félix was pleased with this mark of recognition, but he failed to receive the medal due to his disabled status. Not important, he told me, "but they are wicked".

Secondly, an envious neighbour made nasty comments to him about what he had been buying a while sponging on the State. Félix's intense aggression and guilt were also directed at me because he had not told me that he had bought it. His psychic space was incapable of containing these narcissistic wounds and his depression. Félix committed suicide. A real suicide this time: Ambulance, resuscitation, and hospital. He survived and resumed his analysis sessions. He had wanted to die. He had had the unthinkable before him: loneliness! Do you know what loneliness is like? In his loneliness he read and reread the same book endlessly (The Two Sorrows of General de Gaulle) and listened to the same record ("White Roses": the story of a child that goes to see its mother in hospital when she has just died). The dying mother, the sorrowing father.

The act of suicide, focussed on aggression and guilt which were no longer a game, was necessary so that Félix could finally talk about his depression and the infinite sorrow that he felt. These were the inadequacies of his life, his unknown grandparents and himself. He could then express his guilt for committing suicide *against* me. Our work took a new turn. I remember how a word played an important part. Félix said that his bosses had lacked consideration for him. I commented to him that from now on he could consider himself. Consider his "state of mind", as he called it, but also have some consideration for himself. He projected much less.

His relations with his neighbours and particularly with his son-in-law improved greatly as the years passed and what he had lacked finally emerged: humour.

About a year before we separated, while preparing for the separation, he returned to the astonishing scene which had left such a mark on him. A woman, a nurse, was bending over a dying patient. He had relived the scene when his mother-in-law died in hospital. He did not want to visit her, just as he had not wanted anyone to visit him when he was in hospital. Despite his fears, he did go to see her shortly before her death and relived the scene of the nurses around the dying woman. A fantasy, both attractive and threatening, had become fixed in his mind- woman and death, always denoting the theme of the baby dying in its mother's arms; an inverted fantasy in the song of the white roses, but with the same meaning- Mater *dolorosa*.

We ended our work by mutual agreement. Félix went happily away on holiday. A few years later he managed an operation for a trivial case of hiatus hernia. Finally he had what he wanted: a stomach disorder. He had prostate complications (due to the antidepressants, the doctors said, but he was no longer taking them) then complications with bleeding (the result of his former alcohol dependency?). He died, as he secretly wanted to, in a nurses' arms.

Treating so many hypochondriac patients took away many of my certainties, but created some others. Few patients have fascinated me so much. Félix taught me a lot. Although it is true to say that his hypochondriac symptom appears not to be symbolic, it cannot be considered as completely without a history and incapable of connecting to the patient's representative world. What led him to change was first his split between hypochondria and hyperactivity. Then his depression – inverted hyperactivity – which I experienced before, and often instead of, him. The most important thing was that I was an accepting maternal agency (e.g. for the suicides) and a reliable paternal image. I think the process we went through together enabled him to live for many years with some peace of mind. He was interested in his own psyche and hardly ever missed a session, except for his "real suicide". It is remarkable that the development of his borderline personality neurosis went hand in hand with the slow disappearance of his hypochondria. Should we question its role?

What was it protecting him from? I do not believe that Félix's death occurred because he had "recovered" from it, as a colleague suggested to me one day. I believe that his cathexes were displaced onto his conflict problems, which removed the hypochondriac imperative with which I never concerned myself and paved the way for an infinitely happier affective life. "Recovery" from the hypochondria was merely a collateral effect, as Freud said. And Ferenczi.

Chapter 6

PSYCHOGENIC POST-TRAUMATIC PAIN

Murmuran con dolor su desconcuelo
(Murmur their despair in pain)
Quevedo

"PSYCHOGENIC" LUMBALGICS

I now want to turn to a category of patients who have been what I might call my "masters in dolorology". These are lumbalgics who are described as "psychogenic" by somaticians and are also post-traumatic. They haunt pain clinics and consultations in large numbers. They are prototype patients for several reasons:

- They present with a "pure" form of physical and also psychic pain;
- They are a model of traumatic neurosis but also share something of the other two psychogenic modes, the hysterical and the hypochondriac;
- Finally, they stimulate consideration of the nature of pain, the invasion it involves and the grief

it causes and therefore consideration of the psychotherapy that can be offered to all patients in pain.

I was asked, no doubt due to my dual origins (I had been a somatician and became a psychoanalyst) to take on some cases called "psychosomatic" which I did not always like to refuse. Yet it was with great reluctance that I yielded to urgent requests from rheumatologists to help them treat a particular category of lumbalgic patients. To be precise, these doctors had admitted with commendable honesty that they were often compelled to reject these patients despite wishing to treat them effectively. They wanted to understand why and wanted to learn to act differently. This rather strange situation caused me to agree to their suggestion and work with them for a few months. I remained in that department for thirteen years despite the demands of my other activities because the experience proved to be fascinating.

For once the specialists were not calling on another specialist for a second opinion or specific additional information but for themselves. The attitude of the doctors intrigued me as much as that of the enigmatic patients who were defeating them. Not having much idea of how to handle them, I decided to behave just as I did towards my usual patients.

These were patients in pain without any organic lesions and with no apparent reason for suffering. In the majority of cases they had had an accident, often a quite minor one, and since that time developed incurable lumbar pain.

I saw hundreds of them. The conversations proceeded in the normal pattern of psychoanalysis, non-directive, non intrusive and preferring to listen attentively to the patient's discourse. The patient's imagination can then express itself spontaneously and associatively, far from the constraints imposed by the answers required for a medical questionnaire.

Amazingly, although the patients behaved instinctively as if it were an ordinary psychological conversation without any surprise at its method and were quite happy to talk when simply prompted by an "um" at the beginning, they never asked me who I was or why I did not examine them.

The parachutist's story

> I have been in pain since an accident at work, here across the kidneys. I had to put a very heavy engine on the floor. I saw that the bench was greasy. I called a workmate who told me to get lost. Irritated, I climbed onto the bench ... I really did see that it was greasy. I pulled the engine. I slipped and fell and my kidneys hit the edge of the bench, there, right across. I have been in pain since then. That's it!

Encouraged by my sympathetic silence, he began his "story" again, still insisting that he had seen that the bench was greasy, made a few general remarks and then told the story a third time. Then he gave me some details of his previous life. He was hyperactive, never stopped, worked hard. He detailed his activities and returned to the accident, which he again recounted. Then he stopped talking and reflected. In a more hesitant voice he said:

- "Perhaps it also comes from parachuting.

- You were a parachutist?

- Yes! I did about thirty jumps, twelve of them in operations ... One day I fell into a swamp, my mates were at the edge and it made them laugh. But I sank up to here (pointing to his waist). They were alarmed and went to find a rope, then formed a chain and pulled me out just in time ..."

He stopped, hesitated, stuttered a little ...

- "I have to tell you, Sir, that I have never had much luck.

- You have never had much luck?

- No. There were a lot of us. We were brought up by neighbours, child-minders, various women... My mother liked a good time... My father worked. On my way to school in the morning I sometimes saw my mother lying on a pile of rubbish, dead drunk, with her dress up."

He repeated the gesture of passing his hand over the back of his waist. Across the kidneys, therefore.

This fragment of conversation is quite typical of this type of patient, as we shall see later. By calling them "psychogenic", the somaticians had detected a "psy" origin in the aetiology of their disorders. I therefore expected to find certain characteristics which even then psychosomaticians had described in detail in the people consulting them: lack of imagination and the associative function, operative thought and essential depression, in short a dull, poor-quality delivery and stilted thought. This was not the case. Another difference was that psychosomatic patients presented with an organic lesion but had little or no cathexis of the painful aspect of their syndrome. Whereas although the lumbalgics could not show rheumatologists the expected somatic lesion, they appeared to be united in a pain that filled the whole void. I had not expected them to regale me with a discourse that was so dense, rich, spontaneous and above all expressive. Expressive of the excessive pain which disabled them but was not accepted by the somaticians due to the absence of a causal lesion. Logic caused them to be rejected, which intensified their complaints but reduced their credibility. Something was there inside them, ready to speak and yet silent and unable to express itself other than through a regressive complaint: "It hurts! It hurts!" I had the impression of opening the floodgates or rather of being present at the opening of the floodgates that my attitude of passive listening had led to.

The discourse of lumbalgics shows an extraordinary and rare intuition. They have the ability to tell the story of their lives and to say from the start what one would only expect to see emerging after some psychotherapy. They have an amazing capacity to make connections and condense the recital: for example, in the case mentioned above the connections between several traumatic events (current back trauma, trauma of military service, childhood trauma), and then to weave the fabric of repetition. They can also condense through a host of small details out of which emerges, for example in the case I have quoted, their fate: "I have never had much luck", or their sensitivity to situations of abandonment (his mother, then his mates in the army and at work who let him fall). All that in the first conversation. A psychoanalyst could not fail to be attracted and clearly the attraction was reciprocated. But how could a lumbalgic meet an analyst outside the hospital?

I was also struck by the contrast between the often rather sad and disillusioned attitude they showed and the proliferate insistence of their words, which shed light on a world that I shall now try to define, at least in some aspects. It is important to say at this stage that when I presented these aspects to the rheumatologists, their attitude of rejection gave way to a positive and even enthusiastic investment in these patients who were now so fascinating. Here they are:

1. First of all the existence of a very rich affective world marked wholly by eagerness and a voracious search for affection, which explains the ease of contact. We might wonder why subjects who are so obviously lacking in and needing affection could contrive to be rejected, but this often happens, both in their private life and, as we have seen, in their relationships with doctors. However, the ambivalence expressed by these patients about the central figures in their lives (spouse, boss, doctor...) whom they saw as both good and bad, against a background where aggression was both affirmed and denied, helps us to understand.

2. The openness to the imagination is the second important feature. It involves a description of a fantasised anatomy and physiology bearing little or no relationship to reality and fostered by the phantasmagoria and inner world of the patient, who contains in his own body the theatre in which his anxieties and fears are played out. This imaginary anatomy-physiology, this corporal anxiety connection, encounters the anatomical-physiological world of the clinician. It uses the same words but with quite different meanings, and

is imbued with the patient's anxiety problems. These are two different languages, quite foreign to one another. What lumbalgics say through the channel of their back pain is quite different from back pain itself. But it is not the discourse of the hysteric or the hypochondriac.

3. An encounter with the subject's history: after what I have just said, it is not surprising that the history of the subject's disorder, as told by him in his fantasy-filled language, should coincide with his personal history from the beginning. Consequently, when the chronic lumbalgics were free to talk openly and endlessly repeated their recitals of the accidents that had befallen them, they suddenly began telling a different story, with deep emotion, from an apparently insignificant detail that opened the floodgates: of a trauma before the trauma, the original trauma associated with their early lives. This was the general pattern:

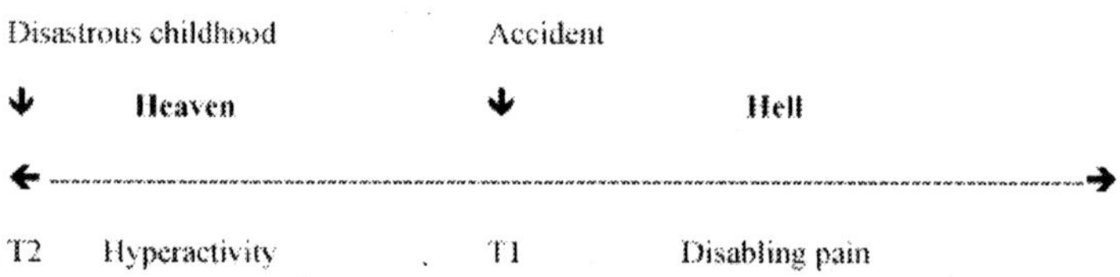

They had had a disastrous early childhood (this was so common that the head of the department where I worked had christened them "Emile Zola types"!), scarred by death, mourning, early separation, abandonment and indescribable distress associated with a chronic lack of affection, incapable of consoling the original distress of the new-born. All these terrible conditions constitute a long-term traumatic situation, not an isolated trauma. This situation had not prevented them from constructing a "Heaven", a period of happiness characterised by hyperactive functioning and recalled in nostalgia. The descriptive force of their discourse made it easy for me to picture this hyperactive happiness. They were nice people, respected by their neighbours and their superiors. They were handymen or gardeners, helped everyone and never stopped. Their recital was lively, entertaining and descriptive. This was "before" the accident. The "after" period was the "Hell", the painful hell of back pain which stopped all their activities.

These patients do not have any hysteria or anxiety (apart from their present anxiety due to the disability and inactivity) or depression in the real sense. There is only the pain, the incurability (often triumphant) of the pain and above all the endlessly repeated complaints associated with it. There is no organic lesion significant enough to be causal among these talkative, interesting, fascinating and eager patients.

We are faced with a pure culture of physical pain, a symptom incorporating its whole meaning and taking it to the limits, an extreme symptom, at the boundary of the physical and the psychic. The hypercathexis of the body in action, muscular effort and external reality (everything happens in hyperactive behaviour) before the accident, then the suffering body afterwards, is suggestive of a rather desertified psyche. Something in these subjects can only express itself through the body, either active and omnipotent or passive and painful.

It is clear why these lumbalgics seemed to me like a kind of prototype of human pain. It was for them that we developed a therapy over the years in the department where I worked (naturally involving the body) and the ideas they inspired led me to organise a special kind of pain clinic at the Neurological Hospital in Lyon.

They are actually prototypes on two levels:

1. Whether psychogenic or not, the pain they feel is real. The fact that it does not respond to conventional analgesics makes this pain a pure phenomenon, so to speak, which can only be treated by working with the patient on the psychic integration of his pain; this is the kind of work that

also has to be done with patients suffering pain due to an organic complaint, particularly when it is resistant to analgesics. So lumbalgics represent a kind of model. One might wonder why neither the medicine of the body nor the medicine of the mind – conventional psychiatry – has made a place alongside, for example, anxiety, depression and syndromes (obsessions, phobias, behavioural disorders, depression etc.) for physical pain as an expression of psychic problems - for human pain, shared by all humanity because it is primal in the destiny of man.

2. They also represent another model: the traumatic model in the psychoanalytical sense. The trauma, eminently repetitive, seeks to reproduce itself. To provoke the doctors a little, I suggested to them that the patients described above were not living in such a painful hell because they had had an accident, but that the accident had been cause because their early disastrous and chronically traumatic childhood would repeat itself one day in an accident ("demoniacally", as Freud said), a true figure of destiny. In short, that the present trauma was an after-shock of another early trauma.

These psychogenic back pain patients are very numerous. They make up a large percentage of the people attending pain centres and clinics. Their development is generally marked by a fixation with the pain symptom and slow deterioration of their condition. As a general rule they never go back to work, although this was their reason for living and their heaven. Some find a surgeon to operate on them and are plagued by worse misery recalling that of their origins.

Back pain as a response

The pain these lumbalgics suffer is due to a trauma. The abrupt appearance of the genuine internal foreign body that it becomes in a psychic economy forms a second trauma which prolongs the original one and joins with it. The result seems to be the after-shock of the traumatic period of infancy.

Although all lumbalgics are different, their discourse is similar in the sense that the four main points which we have already noted in the parachutist patient are expressed quite early on, sometimes even in the first conversation:

- The painful, incurable present, which is a complaint;
- The accident stated to be the cause, despite often being minor, and its circumstances;
- The recent past, hyperactive, wonderful, but lost;
- The ancient past of the disastrous beginnings, experienced in distress.

These points have to be seized on as the recital unfolds, when they are newly expressed. Even if the patients do not connect these four periods, an obscure intuition and a confused feeling of the continuity of their life allows recollection of them. They offer a traumatic model of their pain, in the image of the trauma they believe is responsible: the accident. It is from these points and the signs that emerge from them that what will later become the psychotherapy can be developed.

As I have said, "psychogenic" lumbalgics represent a pure form of physical pain because it is free from any associated somatic lesion liable to have caused it. This absence of lesion is the most direct cause of the lack of understanding between doctors and patients. I often found myself in the position of devil's advocate pleading a difficult case, because there can never be pain without a cause in the eyes of a doctor. The pain and the lack of understanding seemed to me to repeat the situation previously experienced. It was the real reason for my interest in these patients and the fascination they had for me.

I was surprised by the spontaneous recitals of their dramatic early lives given very quickly by these lumbalgics. It is not often that people in hospital for a reason in no way psychological recall such a poignant subject. As we have seen above, these people often do, after a slight hesitation or stammer marking their emotion. It is the emergence of an affect which is initially unobtrusive but then close to tears. The moment has to be captured because it provides a profound understanding of the complaints and pain which they are suffering now, in the department, and which they previously suffered in their earliest infancy, the original misery and distress. This misery represents that of the newborn, the primal *Hilflosigkeit*. This distress is common to all newborn babies. It is due to the physiological immaturity of the human race and demands care to ensure survival and a certain quality in the maternal presence (and also absence), so that the psyche can develop and the humanisation of the child can begin. I shall not enlarge here on the hazards of the early relationship between a baby and its mother; this is discussed in another chapter. But we can say now that a good relationship of this kind involves mutual understanding. In failing to find this with the doctors responsible for curing his pain, the lumbalgic repeats the original situation, the lack of consolation and the same lack of response from those around him. He also repeats the situation of passivity and impotence of the first periods of life, when outside help was needed. The physical and mental pains are added. Although they must also exist in the distressed baby and we imagine that in a form unknown to us they accompany the cries, rage, anger, hatred and violent reactions testifying to the despair of the abandoned, suffering baby. I have described all these sensations as primal affects. These affects have not found a meaning and have not been symbolised but have left what I have called "amnesiac traces" susceptible to physical or behavioural, and also painful, discharges. Although this baby's suffering can be imagined, it is difficult to imagine everything that it has lacked which should have been there. Positive traumas, negative traumas and early narcissistic wounds have left traces which will one day re-emerge and make the subject traumatophilic.

After the accident the subject can no longer act. He can only react to a now internalised object; the pain was hypercathected as was the activity. His final act is the accident which may represent a fusion with the primal object. The accident is the end of an era, a (new) betrayal by the object.

Hyperactivity and repetition

Repetition of an affective and traumatic experience is not surprising. It is what happens in any psychic organisation. But we should not forget that it was on the subject of traumatic neurosis that Freud emphasised repetition. The expression of the experience is itself repetitive and even tedious. Treating these patients involves listening attentively to their endlessly repeated laments, which feed their nostalgia by going over and over their memories. But occasionally, new memories are discovered that are valuable through the spark they evoke in the psyche, tenuous evidence of possible processing. One needs a finely-tuned ear! The lumbalgic repeats everything: the circumstances of his accident, the descriptions of his various pains and his lamentations and regrets for his lost self-worth.

One might think that during the happy period of hyperactive heaven, the repetition had "forgotten" to affect the future lumbalgic. I am inclined to think that it manifested itself in a different way. This rather frenzied hyperactivity is not considered pathological nowadays. It is even often desired. It seems to me to be a frenetic and vigilant defence of the anti-cathexis of the infantile passivity. It can be seen as the anti-cathexis in activity of what was previously experienced passively in impotence and distress. The repetition takes the form of compulsive action, a true repetitive vibration always to be reactivated. The need for it seems to be more important than its content. The ego appears to have attempted to divert the power of the compulsion (*Wiederholungszwang*) to transform it into pleasure and move towards connection and has partially succeeded. But the process expends energy and is fragile, even though many personalities function like this for a long time, some even forever. This is not the case with our lumbalgics.

A large quantity of narcissistic libido is cathected in what is the exact opposite of the previous situation of impotence, distress and pain. The constant fear that it will repeat itself is another means of repetition. The thing that is feared and constantly guarded against finally arrives in the traumatic form of the accident. Then comes the symmetrical opposite of the rather maniacal, omnipotent hyperactivity. It is the lumbar pain and the feeling of impotence and dependence, equally over-cathected and expending of energy.

The accident represents the external cause of a problem for which I have just given some internal motives. The patient sees it as the only reason for his misfortunes, describes it in great detail and frequently returns to it with a sort of fervour. So much so that an animated scene is built up in the mind of the psychiatrist as he listens, but one which seems frozen in repetition. Once again, it is important to pay attention to the minor variations, if any, the hesitations, slips of the tongue and particularly the associations. These small psychic events that occur when an affect emerges, have much to say about the conditions of the accident and sometimes a certain unconscious participation, or at least a decline in the patient's normal vigilance.

For example:

- "I had noticed that the road was wet and it was still raining. I had seen somebody coming from the right at the crossroads. I overtook a motorist who was annoying me, I braked sharply, skidded and the guy went up my backside, he was North African. I don't like North Africans ... (*hesitation*) ... I wonder how it happened! (*he gave me a puzzled look and I gave him an interested one*)."

Hard to say more in so few words. The patient himself was amazed that his experience had not enabled him to foresee the accident and prevent his failure to act. I often said to myself that what these small initial conversational fragments told us was in may ways similar to what can be perceived before analysis during a preliminary talk. In this case, the intangibility of an exchange of looks that must be called pre-transferential was the starting point for a particularly productive period of therapy.

The accident was not causal, as believed by the patient and refuted by the doctor, but it contained a wealth of information and its recital was a true condensation. So the patient was partly right. The associations it yielded told us about his psychic state at the time of the accident and during the period preceding it. It was an abrupt conjunction between his internal and external worlds and merged his various time frames. Many aspects of his psychic situation before the accident emerged, indicating – without constituting a causality – that fragility had developed in the defence mechanism built up and a breach could cause the whole edifice to collapse. This fragility revealed the limits of a defence as monolithic as hyperactivity but also showed against what it was erected. It could be worry about a promotion or change of job or the desire for a child, often a son, to do well in a difficult and important exam such as the baccalauréat ("I wanted him to do better than me!"). It could be the completion of a new house or the start of it; anything that interrupts the continuity of life, or challenges it.

The words continued, repeatedly:

- "I can't even carry a bucket now",

and it was only necessary to ask why this was so important for the discourse to become more complex and sometimes poetic:

- "I am a wreck in a miserable skin!"

It could be remorse associated with the maternal or paternal imago:

- "I should have listened to my father and gone into the army."

Strong affects, therefore, on tenuous fantasies. They had to be picked up to help them to blossom. The seed of elaborative work was there. This work was twofold: firstly, elaborative enlargement of a shrunken psyche channelled by the eroticised pain, and secondly, mourning for all that the patient had lost. In essence the trauma lent itself to repetition rather than elaboration, although we could not fail to see an attempt at elaboration in the repetition.

In addition, and we shall see the importance of this later, the recital of the accident contained something hallucinatory and hyperrealistic which registered in the mind of the listener. In other forms of traumatic neurosis this constantly reiterated recital performs the role played by the screen memory in more conventionally neurotic mechanisms. Not that these two processes of the human psyche should be considered as opposites: they are more like the two ends of a chain that contains many others. I glimpsed a meeting point and even the possibility of treatment inspired by our normal practice. A reason for optimism.

Intergenerational transmission

A number, that of a particular age, sometimes comes up in one of the first conversations and this is rather surprising because it introduces precision into the tenor of the discourse. It is the age reached by a relative, generally the father or mother but it can be someone else, at the time of a - generally unhappy- event. It then also proves to be the age of the patient at the time of the lumbar trauma. Here are two striking examples:

The man with two ages

I noticed the facility in the French language of a young man who told me that he had been born in Algeria. His accent was that of a region of Northern France. He was born in 1936. His father, born in 1900, went into the army when he himself was less than a year old. His mother left him to be brought up largely by his paternal grandfather, who was a "strong man", authoritarian, and was very well known in the district.

In 1940, therefore when aged 40, his father left for France and the war. He was taken prisoner and nothing was heard of him for a long time. His grandfather decided to "look after the inheritance" and manage the farms that it comprised. His mother arranged a divorce, remarried, had other children and lost touch completely with her eldest son.

A few years after the war when he was still very young, only 13 years old, he wanted to go in search of his father, who did not return to Algeria after his release and settled in a small town in the North. He wanted to get to know him:

> - "In Algeria the father is sacred. He has the right to disinherit you seven times. He can take a castle from you. I was 15 years old – in fact I am dead.
> - ?
> - In fact I was 13 years old and did not have the right to travel alone, even with permission from my legal guardian."

He explained: One of his cousins had died of typhoid. He registered his own death at the town hall and took his identity and age, which enabled him to travel alone. With the consent of his grandfather, the Cadi, in front of witnesses according to Algerian custom, he left. He would never reach the city where his father lived. He stayed in a city very close by,

> - "I did not know the language", was his excuse.

He was taken in by a farmer who brought him up "as his own son" and from then on led the life of a European. He married a European woman. He had children with her and gave them "international" names. He worked and earned a good living (he had a job that involved lots of travel).

Two extraordinary accidents then occurred:

When his real age was 40, he had an accident which he himself described as inexplicable. He fell from a height onto his head and also had lumbar trauma. He gave up his job for some time because of his back pain and vertigo, then went back to work against his will at his boss's request.

When he was 40 for the second time (the age of the cousin and his own in his adopted status), he had another accident, just as inexplicable.

- On a bend, I saw the house, I saw the garden, I saw the wall... I crashed into it."
And a curious slip of the tongue:
- "It gave me a shock added to *my previous accidents*.
- ?
- I mean my previous accident."

In this story in which the inheritance is at stake, many things are not transmitted: The inheritance itself was "kept" by the grandfather, Algerian culture was replaced by European culture. Finally, the contact with the father did not take place, and never took place, despite the child's wishes. The father could not leave a memory (a father can disinherit you).

But one thing has been transmitted, just one: the age of the break and the need for it. The age of 40, marking the departure of the father forever. The age of 40, marking the son's break, twice. As the slip of the tongue reminds us, there was also another break much earlier, the separation from the mother.

This case is a perfect example. Several points are significant. Firstly we note the absence of psychic suffering in the patient before the first accident. Then, when we examine the quality of what is transmitted between father and son, as represented by the break, we notice that nothing of the father's history appears in the son's symptoms, the accidents and pain. The need for transmission is much more important that its content, which is just a hollow, non-symbolic symptom that at the time (1980) I suggested calling the "chrone".

Inherited back pain

M. B. was hospitalised for back pain which proved to have no clinical basis. He felt the pain for the first time at work, with a feeling of being paralysed. The doctor he consulted did not prescribe rest from work (non-recognition). While mowing his lawn a few days later, he felt increasingly violent pains and gave up work. I saw him seven months later, still off work.

During the conversation he complained about the various bosses he had had who had never appreciated him.

> - "Four years ago (he assured me) in the army I was hospitalised after a blood serum and was told it was my nerves. And in the night I had an intense, horrible anxiety crisis, I was woken up by an acute pain. I couldn't move, I was afraid of being paralysed".

He was then 20 years old. At the time of the back accident which put him in hospital, he was 24. He then talked about his childhood. His mother had him at 17. She was "maimed by the labour". She had an injured spine: "a drunken truck" crushed her between the pavement and the wheel.

M. B. never knew his father. He was soon collected by his grandparents. His mother had to work. She continued working for three years and at the age of 20 had her accident. Then I learned that at the age of 24 she had had twins by a man from whom she was later divorced.

M. B. returned to his first anxiety episode.

> - "It was at night and I was alone. My wife had just had a baby. She was at the maternity hospital. The walls revolved. I called the doctors. My spine was paralysed down to the pelvis."

The "chronological" inheritance in this case was a double one. What the mother suffered, first at 20 and then at 24, was experienced by the child as a catastrophe. And it was at 20 and then at 24 that he too cracked, without any obvious cause in the spine and pelvis. He did not really know this, but made me aware of it.

In this example the trauma was transmitted from one generation to another by reproducing the mother's symptoms: the pelvis and spinal column. This unconscious identification from body to body was coupled with another capture of the problem of the mother: abandonment anxiety which made him aggressive, depressive and dependent. The somatic symptoms were not the end of the transmission. M.

B. had also inherited from his mother a form of distress accompanied by a feeling of being haunted and even of paralysis ("my spinal column was paralysed ...") that she must also have experienced during her accident.

In psychogenic back pain patients, the current pain reactivates an old unsatisfied demand. There is then a reorganisation around a wound in a psyche previously inhibited, reawakening the strong requirement for care which had previously been transformed into hyperactivity. The lumbar area acts as an algogenic and erogenous zone, burdened with a powerful need for satisfaction.

The strength of the repetition is more intense than the strength of the satisfaction. What kind of satisfaction might this be? The patient is back in the same unsatisfying situation as at the beginning of his life. He asks questions that his doctor cannot answer any more than his mother once could. The sensation of pain demands love but the patient is only given rejection. Impotent, he makes the doctor impotent as the mother once was, re-establishing the old relationship and perpetuating it, rediscovering the past.

The affects they experience alert us. We understand their imperious demands but they make it impossible for us to satisfy them. This is why their doctors are angry. Pain is a constant presence in the stranger within them and the psychic processing that that involves. Something was expelled in the hyperactivity which has surprisingly returned in the form of trauma, without warning or preparation, and bypasses the defences. We have to understand the reality of the repetitive situation and the need for it and sacrifice our desire to cure. We have to accept the difficult relationship established by the patient, should we call it transference?

These patients ask us for the impossible:

- They make us experience what they have undergone;
- They want to relive what they have undergone;
- They are secretly asking us to do what their mothers did not do. To be the ideal mother whom they never knew.

What to do?

I shall now describe the case of a patient suffering post-traumatic but not spinal pain who shows the extent to which the repetition can assume the demoniacal form given to it by Freud. The repetition of traumatic accidents in this patient is impressive. We shall see that - like his lumbalgic brothers - he represents a model and an example, enabling us to imagine an answer to this question.

VICTOR, A PURELY PSYCHOGENIC CASE

Was he a hypochondriac? Yes, because he did not seem capable of expressing anything but his pain, forever and ever. But then he told us his life story and talked about a traumatic neurosis.

Victor came to attend a pain clinic at Lyon Neurological Hospital for chronic pain sufferers run exclusively by psychoanalysts. He was tall, strapping, likeable and voluble. He had hardly sat down before embarking in an attractive Algerian French accent on the monologue that he continued for years:

- "I stopped sleeping thirty years ago. A dog jumped up at me. I didn't see it. It was all white. I was on military service. I fell. My head and my knees hurt. I have insomnia, adult asthenia and chronic fatigue. I have nightmares, with blood."

This was all after an incident that occurred in Algeria during the war. Before that he was fine, hyperactive and afraid of nothing except blood. Since then, during his insomnia, he had recalled and relived his traumatic scene, with nightmares and bleeding. This was the account of the incident that he gave me early in our first conversation and repeated in that same conversation and then, innumerable times over the years. It was the first traumatic scene. There would be others.

He was overworked, driving an ambulance and delivering letters for eighteen hours a day. One evening he went into an Arab house with a letter. The courtyard was surrounded by rooms: the bedrooms of the Muslims. There was total silence. He called out but the women did not come out. They never came out "because of their religion". Still silence. A big white dog jumped on him from behind without first barking. Victor fell onto his knees and head and remained unmoving, paralysed and terrified. The women then came out from all sides, surrounded him and spoke to him. They repeated an Arabic word: *Khela'a*. It means, he told me: He has been frightened. He repeated the word *Khela'a*; he has been frightened, several times.

I was astonished by the word "frightened". It was fright that Freud referred to on the subject of traumatic neuroses when the unprepared ego is overwhelmed and struck down, and cannot defend itself by either anxiety or psychic elaboration. The Arabic word *Khela'a* also surprised me by Victor's cathexis in it. He repeated it with something resembling delight. I noted the different ways he pronounced it. Victor pervaded my mind as he repeated his recital of the scene. Then he suddenly summed it up in two remarks: "Pain, pain, sleep!" and "I still remember the past". These two short phrases, again repeated throughout the treatment, are important. They describe the reality of a memory which can only be expressed with difficulty through language. I would find out that Victor remembered but would only gradually have access to his memories. It was a speechless memory which, unlike that of hysterics, blocked out reminiscences, or only knew of a chronic one, pain. Pain interacting in the other short phrase with sleep. No discharge could soothe the excitation of that pain. It knew only the resolution of sleep.

The two-stage picture that he presented is typical of the trauma patients who come to pain clinics for treatment: a hyperactive paradise, then an incurable physical pain caused by a minor physical trauma or even, as is the case here, by a facilitation not accompanied by physical injury. And yet the body which appears to be trapped in the traumatic moment has garnered a painful memory, incurable from then on. We have seen that this is what happens in some back pain sufferers called psychogenic. But Victor's problem was more complex.

Before the account of the second scene which he gave me several months later, I had some details of his life. There were fourteen children in the family:

- "Seven dead, four living ... and three sisters" ...

A poor family in Algeria: work, work! His father was a farm labourer and Victor always worked in the fields. In 1944, during the war, he showed great heroism, volunteering for all the dangerous missions. He then joined the police and went through the Algerian war, always taking risks. ("I do not fear death or danger", he often asserted.) It was at that time that the incident with the dog took place.

My contacts with Victor were very strange. Locked in his pain, the recital of his pain and the recital of the trauma initiating his pain, he left little scope for his interlocutor. He was both exhausting and engaging and I was charmed by the strange, voluble sadness that he poured out at every session.

The imperfect, the tense preferred by Victor, denoted a past irrecoverably lost. It was a tense of nostalgia and regret. The present was only there to refer to the current pain, in terms frozen in a repetitiveness that discouraged all desire to approach it more closely.

The second traumatic scene that he described to me recalls the first in a strange way. It took place in France after he had left Algeria: Victor was standing in a large dustbin at the building where he was the caretaker. All around him women were complaining and claiming space for their rubbish. Victor trampled rubbish underfoot in the dustbin, which swivelled on its wheels. He fell onto his knees and head. The women rushed up and surrounded him, shouting. Victor's painful symptomatology which had never really been soothed flared up again due to this new trauma. I was obviously very struck by the resemblance to the first scene, but not Victor, who remained deaf to my attempts to link them.

I shall not dwell on the third traumatic scene because it is horrible. Chronologically, it occurred between the first and the second, but I did not hear about it until much later. Victor had remained in Algeria at the end of the war to try to discover the whereabouts of a missing female relative. He felt rather guilty about the disappearance which he had been unable to prevent. Guilty in his own eyes, because he had nothing to reproach himself with. In conditions of great danger and "already ill because of the dog", he finally found what he was looking for: a well, women's bodies, blood everywhere ... It was women's shoes worn by a man that had put him on the track.

The fourth traumatic scene was short and sad. It was also recent. A male relative of his was hospitalised. He had a blood disorder. He was lying on his bed having a transfusion. The nurses were all fussing round him.

A fantasy or a scene, insistent: a man, outstretched (a child?) is surrounded by women and the idea is one of danger, suffering, blood and death. A set of signifiers that recurs inexorably in Victor's life and life story. In the third scene things are reversed: it is the women who are dead, the man is standing up. In every case the affect is one of fright or even terror. It is impossible to connect the fright with reality, except in the third scene (the bleeding well) or to understand why the first two scenes of falls changed Victor into a man who suffered and did absolutely nothing except recount them interminably, like punctuation in the story of his life, also interminable.

I was struck by Victor's undeniable passion and satisfaction. Happy to talk, he would brook no interruptions, which he took to be disparaging of his pain. He even took trivial requests for details badly.

Faced with Victor, my mind worked furiously, particularly around the word Khela'a repeated so complacently, not always in the same way. Pronounced as Victor did occasionally: *Khla*, the word means: void. Victor's usual pronunciation, *Khelaa*, is incorrect. I imagine that he meant: *Khela'a* (with a letter *'a* difficult for Europeans to pronounce). Recollections of my earlier Arabic literature studies and the dialect of my native country gave me the meaning "he is undressed", but, as later confirmed to me by Arabic speakers, the word also means "he has been frightened", as Victor had intended. More precisely: he has frightened, because the subject is the dog; or as a noun: terror, fright.

So Victor repeated his pain and its expression, the words of his pain: complaint. As if the pain were not repetition enough, he also repeated the traumatic scenes and the recital of the traumatic scenes. He also repeated the areas of the pain (head, knees) and the conditions when the pain occurred (the falls).

No affect can find the perfect representation to describe it and this disparity or gap contained the essence of the man: the need to connect, the revival of the desire and the freezing of the thought. It was to the "helpful person", the "clever person" (Freud 1895*a*), through maternal seduction, that he once again responded, externally, to what remained internally of a psyche ready to live.

Strictly speaking the original trauma for him was not sexual; but in that overburdened family, surrounded by deaths, births and money problems, we can imagine that his childhood was difficult, neglected, lonely and marked by abandonment, distress and dereliction. In short, a long-term traumatic situation with too many stimuli and too few discharges, adapted to the conditions and therefore forming a structure.

Victor did not talk equally about the two phases of his life when telling his life story. There were two periods and two origins. The first, operative and hyperactive, was scarcely mentioned. He was always busy (work, work). He was obliging and loyal and always had things to do, either for himself or others ... and he could do anything. The second period, that of the invasive pain, had its origins in the initial traumatic scene. As I listened to Victor, I recalled Ferenczi's brilliant idea about the clever baby, its mastery and its disarray. After the trauma suffered by the baby, a split occurs between a painful and potentially destructive part and an omniscient and insensitive part.

In Victor the split was one of time, with the two phases of hyperactivity and pain. The early trauma produced a surviving violence, similar no doubt to that described by J. Bergeret (1973), a violence felt physically. It was understandable that this violence had been anti-cathected in his body (hyperactivity) and his behaviour.

The clinical course of pain is a negative one. We can see this in Victor. As D.W. Winnicott said:

> "It is easier for a patient to recall a trauma that to remember that nothing happened when it could have happened." (Winnicott, 1974)

We might perhaps add, "should have", as Freud said about Elisabeth.

There are various reasons for the staunch operative hyperactivity of the first of the two stages. It involved intensive anti-cathexis of the destructive drive towards the mother (guardian of the destructiveness towards her), enabling him to avoid expressing the affects of hatred, retaliation and revenge. This helped to preserve his self-esteem, supplied the stimulus necessary to his life and allowed him to regain (or gain) control, mastery and, to a degree, renarcissisation of the ego in omnipotent activity. It involved keeping up a constant defence against any affect and representation of an object kept indistinct. The subject, he himself, functioned only in the present.

In the second period, the pain phase, there was the paradox of a situation in reverse that achieved the same objective: no affect that might be a reminder of the previous feelings of impotence and distress. The change from actively to passively directed drives embodied in inactivity and pain created a system that saved energy and was more effective. In this system stimulus was pain and discharge was also pain. There was little or no room for other affects, apart from a dark hinterland of triumph and defiance: "You will never cure me!" emerging occasionally with obvious delight. These patients often remind us of melancholics or hypochondriacs because they make us sense a fragment of the object, dead, incorporated and buried. But anyway, surely the hypochondriac is a rather self-satisfied melancholic?

Many patients in chronic pain, including Victor, have no expressed or conscious sense of guilt. The action or the pain removes it by different means. As Freud said (1923), they have "a sense of guilt which finds satisfaction in the complaint and does not want to give up punishment through suffering ... But this sense of guilt is silent for the sufferer ... the patient feels ill, not guilty."

In these patients, as in the mourner and the melancholic, the traumatic invasion or mourning is relative in the sense that its potential pain level must be understood as symptomatic of a previous psychic organisation. The patient only blames his pain, but the analyst makes connections and can think otherwise. In cases like Victor's, we are justified in reviving the old idea of traumatophilia to glimpse what is traumatic about a trauma. Things are breakable only when they have become fragile.

I see the pain as a primal, undefined affect, a proto-affect which must be the after-shock of an unnamed, indistinct earlier shock which has not adapted, either to the absent psyche or to the reality which still cannot be grasped by the perceptive apparatus. An indefinable sensation which must be tamed by and for the needs of life. Expressing the pain has a function of appeal.

Michel Fain, quoted by Gérard Bayle (1996) says that if "the normal priority of erotic activity is replaced by the priority of suffering, it then exceeds the integrational potential of the primal masochism". We can say, then, that too much pain kills masochism or limits its soothing function, but also that an excess or residue of pain imposes a masochistic need.

In this case, the self-withdrawal which masochism accomplishes by repatriating the drives to the ego prevents the object being properly established, and even less being lost and therefore being regained. It is the skeleton of an object that has encountered the sad symmetry of a skeletal ego. The subverted masochism, powerless to find the sadistic object, leaves the pain free to exert itself in an autoeroticism of pure endless discharge. It is to be hoped that this autoeroticism has a calming (or rather self-calming) function. Patients in pain sometimes have gestures of infinite tenderness, the gestures of a mother, to caress their internal injury. A dog licks its wounds. The aggression slumbers, sometimes, happily, with the eruption of a sudden rebellious gesture that reveals the smouldering fire: a violent attack on a doctor seen for a moment as a persecutor, seldom organised resentment, sometimes the manifestation of a mental masochism which generally aggravates the situation, leaving little or no way of using it.

The pain is not silenced by expressing the complaints. It is accompanied by silent resignation or dumb accusation. Against whom are they aimed? The complaints are against X. They form a world of torment, outside all representation, and aggravated by the inability to represent an object which has become blurred by its absence. This need for complaint is the discharge of the painful autoeroticism, its masturbation. In the consultation it takes the place of psychism; the affects that it conveys, felt en masse in the pain, search desperately for a meaning. They represent an appeal that remains deaf to any response, by default; an appeal which finds no object, seeks no object, but remains as a witness to the suffering and also as a vestige of a maternal image retained hopefully through the despair.

What is the fate of this painful autoerotic narcissism in a face-to-face consultation and under psychotherapy? It has to be seen as a sudden stopping point or ending that bars the way to an even more serious narcissistic collapse. It constitutes a sounder defence than one might think in its slow dynamic of obdurate repetitiveness. The fear of collapse, breakdown or even annihilation in some cases, is immediate and so dangerous that the patient clings to his defence mechanism. The clinging is anal in nature. This anal function is revealed in the consultation. The patient controls everything. Nothing must be allowed in or out. Nothing bad must happen to him and nothing good either, especially anything new, which would be immediately destroyed. But expressions like "Well OK! If it doesn't make things worse!"

show where the danger lies. In this effort at contention on the one hand and destructiveness on the other, even the ambivalence is frozen, like arm wrestling between two men of equal strength. How to intervene? I have spoken earlier about the survival problems of the therapist. My fascination for the word *Khela'a* is a sign of this, or of my need to function mentally.

A strange phenomenon also has to be understood and accepted: the patient talks to us as if we were him. He invites us in some way to participate in dual autoeroticism and makes us into a double narcissistic mirror image. So often dependent and childlike, he now shows his imperious, autocratic side. He speaks and we must say nothing, having become the double, empathising enough to allow identifications, but not too much. The problem is a complex one. The therapist is wedged between two positions: to survive psychically in the complaints while continuing to listen, and to accept the autoscopic relationship and become the narcissistic double of his patient.

He risks drifting between the two, losing his own boundaries and in his regression experiencing a traumatic state that attacks his personal representative world. He can cope with it by theorising or by moving his thoughts to other fantasies, which is better (for example by being interested in the word *Khela'a*). He can also retreat into an imaginary scene, taking the form of animist ideas to ensure the continuity of his psyche, despite the drift he feels. In the same moment of drift, far from feeling an unrepresentable affect (or anxiety in the face of non-representation, as believed by César and Sara Botella, 1984), the patient puts up with being in pain. The visual element of the face-to-face situation may give better protection than the analysis situation could. The patient keeps his eye on us!

This kind of wavering can be used in the therapeutic relationship. As we shall see, when the language again becomes polysemic it is responsible for reassembling the memory and offering facilitations. This is what happened to Victor, in a transferential incident.

In the midst of his plaintive monologue, he became confused, began babbling and stopped for a moment. I gave him what was probably rather an odd look. I felt something unidentifiable. He saw my look and said:

- "After my first fall I was given *penetrating* radiotherapy" and immediately put his hand on the back of his neck with a gesture of suffering. I cannot remember why I looked at him like that, but I remember my agitation. Our affects crossed. In any case, I penetrated him. Victor moved on to some obviously homosexual fantasies, but then another memory came back to him: the horrific scene of the bleeding well. This opened up two quite different routes to psychic elaboration; the route of homosexuality with its potential for structuring, even though it initially appeared dangerous, and the route of destructiveness and death. For the first time in a session, an uncontrolled affect appeared, an affect outside the usual tenor. Then Victor began associating in ways that introduced new memories:

- "The Arabs have a very sharp dagger [...] I knew one who had killed a man. I never let him walk behind me."

Then he made a slip of the tongue when saying *Khela'a*; he added a feminising ending:

- "She has been frightened."

I took note. Some time later a memory came back to him: he was working on his knees in a field. Suddenly he heard a noise, then nothing, then again. He was very frightened. He would be penetrated. Dagger? Penis? Both? He began speaking in Arabic... behind him, still silence, then a reply. He was saved! In the following sessions many other wartime memories emerged. He talked about a very tough commanding officer:

- I could not stand up, was clinging to a tree. He said to me: 8 days in gaol, unless you have a fever. Fortunately I had a bout of malaria. I liked the officer." (!)

Victor tentatively explored his own psyche. He could not really elaborate the primal violent scene involved in his fall with the dog, but he could decondense it a little and two fantasies emerged: the women who do not move when they are called (but keep being called) and, with the word "penetrating", the daggers, the dog's fangs or the cruel commanding officer, a tough but ever-present paternal figure seemed to be released from the previously all-pervading image of the phallic mother.

The images became livelier. The affect was no longer fully lost in the pain. Victor began wondering why he had gone into the courtyard, which was forbidden ("harem" is one of a family of words from a root that means both sacred and forbidden). The fact that he went was more an indication of the childhood desire (to penetrate the parents' bedroom) than of the need to control by going back over the traces. He could investigate his sense of guilt and the punishment that went with it and, projectively with the officer, his great ambivalence. At the same time a very tentative transference occurred, to be used rather than interpreted.

It is in these circumstances that the defences risk being overwhelmed; when the reunions with the hated object via an almost hallucinatory representation, reactivate a poorly symbolised trace. I used to call this trace "amnesiac" (1974). It is discussed in more detail in other chapters. It is incapable of bringing recall, but it can either create or maintain the immobility of the chronic pain, suspended in repetition, or precipitate the traumatophilic subject into a new traumatic accident.

What paradoxical pain! Born in the inadequacy of the maternal stimulus barrier, creating traumatophilia, it becomes itself a stimulus barrier through the continuous excitation it arouses. Through the failings of this stimulus barrier, for example "the psychotherapeutic incident" related above or the circumstances of the traumatic scenes recounted by patients, we can notice the forms, images and representations which may, when taken up by the language, allow work on psychic elaboration. The recital of the traumatic scene then becomes the screen memory of the poor sufferer, the poor painful ego.

In trauma patients, the inner violence which has not been adequately discharged in the psyche remains close to the perceptive. It is discharged in motility. The over-intense perceptions remain meaningless, fixed in "amnesiac" traces that have not become representations. The child keeps its pain and tries, year by year, to discharge it in action and in a behaviour neurosis. Internal discharge (for example screen memory or neurotic symptom) cannot adequately take place, but external discharge in action is possible. The subject becomes operative, hyperactive, kind and loyal, as Victor was "before". But he is also fragile, possibly traumatophilic, and in this case has a date with a "traumatic moment", an ersatz screen memory previously undeveloped due to the lack of screen or internal scene and projected into the future. What I call the traumatic moment is a conjunction, an explosive encounter between internal and external and between the past and the present. When the trauma awaiting the subject happens, he somehow recognises it. The perception experienced now recalls a perception previously experienced which had kept its power and could not be metabolised. It overactivates him. The screen is now there, on the outside, in the reality which "demoniacally" pounces on the patient as he races towards it. Time is trapped. The past, in almost hallucinatory reminiscence, is repeated in the present. Pain has invaded in an explosion of affects previously forced out.

In the depths of the mortified and now painful layers of the stimulus barrier can be heard, in Victor's case, the survival of an ever-present female mother image, allowing investigation of the vague forms of a father whose killing has not been accomplished. Otherwise, what is the meaning of all the repetitive forms to be seen in Victor's recital of his misfortunes? For example, those knees and that head which by accident in his falls and adventures hit the ground, in who knows what Arabic prayer, the meaning of which escapes us? Or the repetitive silence – of the courtyard, the women, the scene in the fields, the dead bodies in the well? Perhaps we can see a repetitive automatism, but that is not everything. There is also a search for meaning and an attempt at connection. The repetition-encounter between an outside world - which despite everything is representative of the inner world - and the inner world itself, however traumatic it may be, is not merely a conveyor of meaning. It is a participant in the castration and Oedipus complex representations through the language. Although they are still tentative and remote and do not mask the sombre images of the dead child, dead to himself and in the eyes of his mother, they represent hope for the traumatic pain sufferer.

And then? What meaning to give to the physical pain and its enigma? A patient with a painful ego is immature, guilty and innocent. He has turned to another person who has not heard. He may feel blamed and often is. Frozen in his suffering, he is there, in suspension, waiting, in his eternal demands. He is a person in the accusative. He needs a spokesperson to understand and make others understand that the primal pain is associated with life.

Chapter 7

"ORGANIC" PAIN: TORTURE SUFFERED, TORTURE DESIRED

The well being that we usually feel is determined by a combination of sensations and coenaesthaesia that we pay no attention to. But the slightest false note in this reassuring concert alerts us, and we try to translate the information to defuse the anxiety it has aroused. In this way we prolong the stimulus and pain barrier function passed on by the maternal agency, because pain is the enemy.

And yet pain is always there, very close, and we have to learn to come to terms with it. We have to accept vaccination to prevent disease (a different pain). We have to suffer to be beautiful. We have to go out in the cold to school and learn to read and grow up.

The violence which presides over our early lives and seems essential, or fundamental, as J. Bergeret calls it (1984), and the aggressiveness which derives from it, which we have to control to become human, demand from us a process of learning and becoming civilised. The picture of our modern world shows how difficult this is. Man likes, or learns to like, inflicting pain on his fellow man and sometimes on himself. He only discovers pain through illness, injury, trauma or, as I have tried to show, certain psychological predispositions. Sadism and masochism are rife wherever men live, whether on a regional, ethnic, religious or individual level. Violent delinquency is increasing and it almost seems as though today's sexuality has become sadomasochistic.

In the earlier chapters I examined how the presence of pain affects the economy of the individual. I thought it would be interesting to see what happens when pain is suffered against the subject's will in torture situations and extreme situations caused by war. But also when it is desired, for example in the masochists called perverse or when it accompanies some modern practices: tattooing, piercing, branding, deep-in and others.

PAIN INFLICTED

Although I have been given personal accounts of torture, I have based this section largely on a very moving article by J.-C. Rolland, "A tortured man" (1986) written following his relationship with Tito de Alencar. It is essential reading. It shows how extreme abuse destroyed a man, a Dominican monk who was a deeply committed leftist activist in reactionary Brazil.

> The torture was so bad that Tito tried to kill himself in prison by severing an artery in his arm and barely survived. It was in France, after his expulsion, that Rolland met him. The man was not just destroyed; he was a different person, a stranger to himself, a creature of the torturers. Under a compulsive need to talk but unable to do so: his notes written in prison and the words of the spoken language did not allow him to express the inexpressible. Then Tito began reliving his experiences, confusing his hospital room with his cell and the doctors and later the Dominicans who took him in with his torturers, regressing to somewhat dramatised action to better express the unconscious.

> Then he took refuge in delirium. But neither the written or spoken word, nor the repetition acted out, nor the delirium, none of these stealthy recollections, could reorganise his shattered psyche. The stress of repetition combined with the internal demands that urged him to speak remained sterile and were unable to organise in mental elaboration, psychic survival or mere survival. He was already dead, in part and in essence, under the electric shocks and charges (one session lasted from 8 am to 2 pm...); not just destroyed, but transformed. He committed suicide when he seemed to be improving by hanging himself from a poplar tree in a public discharge. A death as pathetic as the ghost he had become.

This extreme example was treated with great skill and depth by Rolland, who analysed not only the internal ravages caused by the torture but also the regressive identification displacement tending to confuse the victim with the torturer. A Russian proverb says that the handle of the knout links the giver with the receiver. In this displacement Tito identifies with the desire of the sadist, feels guilty and thinks he has talked. The external and the internal merge and internal self-excitation takes over from external stimulus. What occurs according to J.C. Rolland is "a very clear dissociation between the immediate consciousness of the facts and a more unconscious internalisation where there is no longer a difference between the torments suffered and desired". In a process that brings our defences and the impossible identification into play, our first instinct is to dismiss this shocking statement. But then we realise that the situation is like a dream, a scene of expression for the id. The valences disrupted by the savage drives no longer have a meaning. Everything becomes desire and that the regression is such that the pain, violently co-excited, finds a horrible satisfaction in confusing its source and its object. "Confusion and guilt come about as the consequences of some disintegration of the internal and external categories," adds Rolland. "The desire is rediscovered in the work ... in the delirious reconstruction of the torture", in other words, in the delirium experienced in France.

No barrier or anti-cathexis can halt the process. To seal the breach opened by physical pain and the goal it produces, Freud refers in *Beyond the Pleasure Principle* to an anti-cathexis capable of acting as a plug, not to calm it but to balance its destructive forces. A "counter-load" which must have an energy. But Freud tells us that only a system which is itself "highly cathected is capable of taking up an additional stream of inflowing energy and ... binding it psychically". This was not possible in this case.

Other torture victims and subjects suffering intense and prolonged acute or chronic pain pressures (such as thalmic pain), defend themselves against the disintegration recognised by Rolland in Tito de Alencar by a phenomenon of dissociation. This is also the case on occasion with people who have experienced unendurable violent psychic traumas. We are bound to recall Ferenczi's split, with part of the ego struck dumb and insensitive and another part trying to control its double. A split which immediately becomes defensive.

> A woman who had been in the resistance during the German occupation and was arrested by the Gestapo and tortured by Klaus Barbie found herself in a very different situation from Tito. She had been active in the resistance, had important responsibilities and although not expecting to be arrested was aware that it was a possibility. She explained that when she was tortured she had to hold out for some time without talking despite her terrible suffering. Then she had the feeling of being split in two. She *saw* herself on the torture table and addressed her torturer in her mind: now you can do what you like, I know I shall not talk!

In her case the dissociation was somehow made use of by her great determination not to talk and then recovered by the narcissistic gain which the heroism of the situation achieved. With the idealism of her cause and the determination she felt, this woman had kept her hopes alive. The events of the war hinted that the Germans would be defeated, which must have prevented her regressing as much as Tito de Alencar. He must have known that he was lost. In his case the dissociation could not produce this defensive split and by merging the agencies it plunged him into confusion and madness.

I have myself treated a number of torture victims, some of them for a long time.

> He had lost his bearings. He had been tortured by the French army, which was trying to find out the names of the FLN leaders in the area, although he was a Messalist (a member of Messali Hadj's party). And later by FLN agents who wanted to find out details of the Messalist organisation, of which he knew nothing because he broke with them when he came to France. In neither case did he have the resources to avoid torture by talking. He showed me the terrible marks on his arms from the torture he had undergone. He felt broken, had lost his political idealism and distrusted everyone, but had been able to regain some balance between structuring cathexes (family, work, cultural development) and the flames of hatred that sometimes flared up in him. He returned to Algeria after independence. I saw him again a few years later in a catastrophic state of breakdown and persecution, seeing conspiracies everywhere. He had found an abiding enemy in the FLN, but his delirious and disorganised musings were directed at all sides. A short stay in hospital and excellent treatment provided by a psychiatrist friend restored his equilibrium to some degree. He was able to leave for Algeria. "I was a wreck," he told me as he said goodbye. He too had been destroyed.

I cannot end this chapter without mentioning other victims of our crazy century. I am thinking of the veterans of the 1914-1918 war and the concentration camp victims. The characteristic that they share is that they never talk about their horrible experiences. Why? Because they are unbelievable or inexpressible, they reply. I noticed that the ex-combatants who came to be prescribed medication on their certificates (article 64 at the time) insisted, "that they had a right to it". They were owed something. When they talked to me, I understood. The horrors they had seen were too remote from the words describing them. Verdun, the Somme, the Chemin des Dames are words stripped of their meaning. We have to imagine bodies carefully piled up in mud 80 cm deep over distances of hundreds of metres to allow horses, carts and troops to pass without getting bogged down, to hear about 400 soldiers mounting an attack and only 4 returning alive but maddened and then being told to go back, or to read "you had to get yourself killed on the spot, anyone who retreated would be shot!" All that to be told at the end of a meal, "please don't talk about Verdun any more!" so they kept silent. And it is only in recent years that the veil has been lifted on the atrocities of the First World War.

But they were alive and were bathed in narcissistic national glory. The physical suffering they endured, the hunger, thirst, cold and wounds, all were set aside because they were alive! War memorials and ceremonies, scars and amputations played their anti-traumatic part. I think this is why Freud believed that a trauma accompanied by an obvious lesion or wound rarely produces a traumatic neurosis. We now know that this is wrong, unless the wound or trauma is accompanied by a good enough narcissistic halo. Again, the anti-cathexis established must be sound and permanent. Someone who loses his job nowadays due to a disability can have a narcissistic breakdown and can be expected to get bogged down in action aimed at improving his pension.

The former concentration camp victims are the most silent. I began a few very cautious conversations with some of them. They began coming to see me on some pretext or other and started talking. When I read Primo Levi, Antelme and others, I recalled the sorrowful, reserved tone they often used. It was a mark of their utterly random struggle for survival against the excessive violence which they could not allow to emerge in either images or affects. A dark and silent memory. With the camp victims, as with the 1914-18 veterans, there was an urge to talk and an inability to do so, unless they were given space for their words and it was the right moment. Many of those I knew seized on it.

One evening a former prisoner from the camps came to ask me to visit him. When I arrived, he talked without giving any reason for more than two hours in a level tone. He proceeded with his recital like a tired storyteller, without interruption and without breaking his rhythm. When he finished we stood up, both silent, and I left. Several years later, I read in a local newspaper article about anniversaries and commemorations that his daughter knew nothing of his past except that it had happened. I was tempted to write to her, but did I have the right? I shall never know why her father asked to talk to me. I have the strange impression that his recital was in colour and so it has remained in my memory, as if the excessive and inexpressible trauma had been conveyed to me in these brilliant colours. That evening the pressure of the internal stimulus had overwhelmed the ex-prisoner. We never saw each other again.

In his book *If This is a Man*, Primo Levi writes shortly after the war expressing the "need to tell others, to make others be involved" as an imperative. We feel the indecency of contact with the horrors of a fearsome testimony in the comfort of our lives, but it is our duty because man's murderous madness seems to have gone beyond all limits and we need to know this.

Apart from this, Primo Levi teaches us many things about pain. Claude Smadja commented on them in *The Evil Being* (1997). He says that his point of view "is limited voluntarily to a psychosomatic point of view" of a concentration camp clinic ... which reveals the ultimate psychic mechanisms developed by men under extreme conditions. He describes two stages. The first traumatic, brutal and violent- the arrival at the camp and the disappearance of all normal points of reference: "in a few seconds we stopped being men". The second stage is the establishment of an operative state and especially a "particular method of handling psychic pain".

I would add that psychic and physical pains were merged.

> "The struggle against hunger, cold, fatigue and blows were the subject of continuous over-cathexis ... Any painful affect became a useless luxury which endangered survival ... The experience of pain and its representative character for the psyche was replaced by an operative system which reduced its intensity and enabled it to be tolerated" (*op. cit.*)

Smadja also notes the antalgic function of this operative state by which the subject cathected everything in the struggle for survival.

Not everything though, because a split occurs, as in any situation of extreme trauma. For example, if the pain was de-cathected in order to survive, a powerful object or sublimated cathexis must have not only persisted, but must have been over-cathected to become the motor of the ability to survive (hope, hatred and above all commitment to a political, religious or other ideal). It was necessary to establish and maintain strong anti-cathexis. The "Muslims" were the ones who had lost this ability and their death came quickly.

The destructive effects of pain are expressed in different ways. The psychic changes caused by the destruction also vary widely. The link made by C. Smadja with Levi's book shows the analogy with what the resistance fighter tortured by Barbie had developed in order to resist: distancing of the sensation of pain and cathexis of her resistance idealism.

The case of Tito de Alencar is an extreme example, as I have said. By crushing his psyche, the methods used against him left him without internal resources, completely passive. He was unable to try to keep or regain an active position by his writings or in a certain sense by his suicide attempt. As we saw, outside help could not revive his annihilated spirit later. His melancholy air and paranoid appearance were just crude forms and the beginnings of the struggle against destruction and the actual suicide, its outcome. At the end of his article J.-C. Rolland muses on the fascination that these experiences can have for us.

PAIN DESIRED: MASOCHISTS

"Fascination": Michel de M'Uzan repeats the word at the beginning of his famous and terrifying article "A case of perverse masochism". He adds "horrified incredulity", and these are the emotions that we feel on reading his account. We can understand why he waited about ten years to publish it. All I can do is refer to the text (1977) and give a broad outline of it to provide an understanding of the picture that we have of a masochist who desired and suffered unimaginable torture. M'Uzan called him 'Mr. M.' or just, 'M'.

> M was tattooed nearly all over with inscriptions revealing his desire to be beaten, debased, sodomised and feminised, and his coprophagy. His right breast had been burned and lacerated with a branding iron, his navel was a crater of molten lead and straps from which he could hang were cut into his back. He had cut off one of his little toes himself with a hacksaw. His rectum was enlarged and there were needles all over his body. His genitals were mutilated and pierced with rings. M described the extremely brutal practices which he underwent when submitting completely to a sadist. He had married his cousin, also a masochist, who among other things hanged herself by her breasts which had butcher's hooks inserted in them. I report this because she seems to have been devoured by her own masochistic needs. She died at 23 of pulmonary tuberculosis, while M., despite the intensity of increasingly cruel practices, somehow managed to live with his perversion without being affected. Although it had began when he was still at school, he gave it up at the age of 45 to 50 and his dreams then returned to

"normal" – erotic, voluptuous, heterosexual and hardly ever masochistic.

The example of the married couple shows that it is difficult to generalise and similar practices can satisfy very different compulsions. M was very much in love with his wife and his masochistic perversion was an addition to a quite normal sexuality, imbued with tenderness, to meet an economic necessity, a need for stimuli associated by M. and also by M. de M'Uzan (after Freud as he tells us) with a genetic factor. It is true that what we know of M.'s childhood hardly sheds light on this compulsion. We can accept the genetic factor (his cousin and wife, and apparently also his father, were masochists), but is this enough to explain M.'s frenzied search for more and more elaborate tortures and greater and greater pain? The hereditary genetic factor is said to have been represented by this need to seek stimulus and a progression from stimulus to pain, then pleasure and finally, but not always, orgasm was then established.

But why would the stimulus be converted into a search for pain? Why could it not find other outlets to discharge and assume more diverse forms? We naturally think of the elaborative possibilities of the psyche, but even if these are not practicable, we know of methods of self-calming other than pain. Mr. M. did sometimes practise them, being capable "of covering distances of up to hundreds of kilometres on foot during his holidays". But it seems obvious that he preferred the perverse erotic and masochistic system that brought him pleasure and orgasm to this solipsist solution, doubtless to satisfy his sexual needs but also because the masochistic practices involved a sadistic partner.

I have been wondering about this: whatever the "exceptional power of the instinct" explained by the genetic factor and his tendency to immediate and total discharge, the mechanism of this extreme masochism cannot be understood unless it is accepted as untameable. That is to say, the physical exchanges with the mother object and the relationship that followed did not allow the purely quantitative to be transformed into mutual understanding. The exchange of pleasure, in short did not bring about the maturing process through which desire is formed and keeps finding new forms and new achievements, never finally completed but always structuring. The mother is complicit in this development through her libidinal cathexis and the anti-cathexis possibilities that she offers to the child. This is the only valid stimulus barrier, one capable of absorbing the traumas and wounds of life through psychic elaboration and making it increasingly complex.

Mr. M. bypassed this development. His thirst for stimulus clearly repelled any stimulus barrier system. But we then have to accept a paradox. Any break in the continuity of the libidinal cathexes, the mother's absence, the non-arrival of the object awaited, anything generating pain, must, by increasing the basic stimulus, have provoked the desire he was seeking, which was ever greater stimulus. What would be distress for anyone else was experienced as an end, or a means of achieving the desired aim, an assumption into pain. In other words, everything I have said about the distressed states too often found in infancy, the early attacks on the ego referred to by Freud in *Moses*, failings of the parental environment that play a part in the aetiology of the main categories of pain - hysteria, hypochondria and traumatic neuroses - makes no sense in the context of the problems of M. and other great perverse masochists; unless it is thought of as a defence.

It appears that in M.'s case the stimulus called up the stimulus in a process of self-acceleration activating pleasure and finally orgasm:

- "At the beginning it hurt, then the erection came. We carried on... the pleasure emerged ... Ejaculation occurred when the pain was strongest... afterwards I simply suffered."

So extreme pain triggered orgasm. It is noticeable that at the precise moment when it was unbearable, M. resembled Tito de Alencar in what Rolland said of him, but with such control over the event that he reached the orgasmic peak. M. de M'Uzan emphasises the point that the fantasy aspect was quite incidental. This does not surprise us because the bypass mentioned above prevents a certain process of psychisation. There is no acting out of fantasies in the torture arrangements set up by M., but there is true programming, M. de M'Uzan tells us. Programming requiring the presence of the sadistic partner, guided like a puppet by the all-powerful masochist to terrifying limits that were not crossed, because: "the sadist always chickens out". So not too many fantasies for M., who had to find inspiration from reading to imagine the torture sessions he wanted to suffer; instead there were affects, contempt for the person applying the torture and above all immense arrogance, a gigantic phallus and pride at being a sort of masochist champion. He only knew one man tougher than himself, "who lived in a cage bristling with spikes". Note that this arrogance cannot be connected only with imagining grandiose narcissism because it was fully justified by the reality of the torture he endured. The apparent triumph masked a desire for abasement of the personality and a need for humiliation which made him accept homosexuality and coprophagy. This was perhaps evidence of the failure of union with the mother and concealed a deep early wound, according to M. de M'Uzan thinks. This brings us back to the discussion on the role of pain.

EXCESS AS AN ATTEMPT AT HEALING

Stoller, in an article entitled "XSM" reports conversations he had with some members of the Los Angeles SM community. Four of these people, heavily into brutal masochistic practices, had suffered serious and painful illnesses from childhood. The need to control the real torment of their pain had led them to accept the suffering and "work through it in their heads", dream about it and transform it into pleasure and then the delights of masochism. Stoller thinks that the more intense the physical suffering experienced during the childhood illnesses, the more intense the need for sadomasochism. He accepts that this hypothesis needs to be confirmed but provides a bibliography that points in this direction and, interestingly enough, this opinion is shared by one of the four people. They were chosen because they practised very hard SM "directed more towards physical pain than master/slave scenes where pain is not hugely important". The conversation reported is quite unbearable and I shall refer to the text without going into detail.

The afflictions of three of these people were: a disabling hyperalgesic vertebral disorder in Norma's case; very severe asthma from birth with repeated emergency treatment and hospitalisation, in Ron's case and violent headaches, vomiting and sensory problems due to migraines or epilepsy in Toni's case. The fourth, Dan, suffered from cystic fibrosis (mucoviscidosis), a condition which required frequent medical attention, unpleasant periods in hospital and very painful daily care, as well as a very short life expectancy.

The conversation – probably recorded – which is conveyed to us has a valuable and illuminating associative spontaneity. It confirms Freud's statement maintaining that only a system that is "highly cathected is capable of taking up an additional stream of inflowing energy and binding it psychically". When submissive, Toni is capable of taking a vast amount of pain. But when as dominatrix her left lip is pierced, as some of them can reverse their roles, she keeps on crying and screaming. Although she says, "it is only slight pain", it is one she finds unbearable. "If the same thing is done to me when I am submissive and I feel docile, it's OK."

Dan has to be in the right mood and then the pain arouses and stimulates him. "Arousal and stimulation are my thing!" says Norma. "But when I don't like something it really hurts me. Lots of things give me pleasure. I cannot describe them as pain, it's pleasure" and "the memory of the pain is really nice". "Otherwise no-one really likes pain", adds Toni.

These sufferers from somatic illness who experienced physical suffering very early in life often began their auto-sadistic or masochistic practices (as we shall see, it is very difficult to define them) at a very young age. The limits that we might imagine would stop them were easily crossed or ignored, as in the case of M., but the starting point was very different. In M.'s case it all began with a primal fact, an intense level of stimulus which found in physical pain an immediate, preferred and therefore cathected form of expression. His stimulus comes from inside and pain gives him if not a meaning at least a channel of discharge which itself becomes stimulus. We can imagine that maternal dreaming of a different quality could have tamed the brutal fact of pain and opened up other more complex, different means of discharge, particularly psychic. Perhaps some people have a violent tropism towards pain, a current which is too strong to be diverted elsewhere. If this is the case pain is not a solution and does not have a function, it is a necessity. Could it again be genetic?

The four masochists of R.J. Stoller are quite different. In their case the pain inherent in their condition comes from the body, therefore from outside; it is not a by-product of the stimulus, it *is* stimulus. By processing the stimulus as pain, M. gained some control and could make himself suffer, which he did very early, as we have seen. Whereas the chronic and often very intense pain of the four sick children forced them into a state of passivity. Etymologically, to suffer is to bear. The habitual if not constant presence of the pain formed a closed, unapproachable world that could not be "worked through" in the sense of *Durcharbeit*, in the affective relationship and emotional exchanges with the parents, however close they were. Pain isolates, and the children had to try to find some way of influencing their experience of pain.

Toni, whose headaches sometimes lasted for three or four days, accompanied by vomiting and tactile hallucinations, would bang her head against the wall, causing nosebleeds, to chase away the "imaginary things" and replace them with something she was sure of. A pain created against one suffered. Then she began to confuse the two. She began to like her migraines, then pain generally and finally masochistic practices. Norma soon began cathecting the physiological pain of menstruation ("it can be used for interesting things") and to cause it, such as by stopping herself urinating. Then she discovered SM quite naturally through auto-sadism (pricking her breasts with needles), causing a dramatic turnaround from passivity to activity, then hard masochism in which the passivity is only apparent. Sadism is only a complement or instrument of the masochist.

Both women talk about their fantasies. They soon emerged when they stayed at home alone instead of going to school because they were ill and their suffering naturally made them masochistic. Their fantasies also represent the beginning of control over a painful reality. Norma's are more inclined to be submissive with a desire for punishment. Toni refers to "psychological masochism": humiliation and degradation, apart from a taste for pain.

Dan, who suffered the most during childhood and had the most frequent serious complications and long periods in hospital, is also the most masochistic of the four (the "best", as Ron said). He explains the why and how of his masochistic journey. His theorising is interesting. The terrible abdominal pain he suffered as a child could last for weeks without respite. "He used to put clothes pegs and clips on his nipples to cause an erotic pain stronger than the other pain." To relieve his stomach, he rubbed it "with all the rest" against the sheets. There followed masturbation without the hands and the pain became a nirvana, an enormous pleasure. After orgasm, the pain returned more strongly (as with M.). The counter-charge or anti-cathexis referred to by Freud to fight against the pain was therefore the pain itself, eroticised. As time passed, Dan cathected this self-inflicted pain more and more for itself as such, and surrendered to harder and harder experiences, demonstrating good imaginative effort, unlike M. When he met Pam, who had not been at all sadistic until then but was seduced by his self-mutilation and genital transformation (nails in the penis, various rings), he began a submissive relationship with her, but remained, apparently, the organiser of his torments. He had a need for pain, an almost addictive need. Ron sums up the situation well: "Some things are done for pleasure and others to manage to live", which clearly shows the two different roles of pain. One is defensive (performing the function of anti-cathexis) and the other erotic, masochistic and necessary like an addiction. This latter possibility raises some questions. Is it a predisposition? People who have suffered or been tortured do not normally become masochists.

We can understand the need in all these subjects to move from passivity to activity and replace the stimulus of the pain caused by the illness with a controlled stimulus, as inflicted by a sadist who is once again only the arm of the masochist. It is difficult to assess the place and function of the fantasies. They dissolve in the inventive world of the masochistic scenes and practices invented. We can see in Dan the continuation of normal sexuality with "girls" and also to some extent with Pam. They had a deep mutual attachment. Dan had also retained an area of sublimation; he was a published poet and looked after sick children.

PAIN AS SURVIVAL

Another cystic fibrosis case is described by Patrick Miller in his article "Pain: a survival therapy" (1999) written about the film "Sick". In the film Bob Flanagan suffers from the disorder and is aware of his short life expectancy, but at the age of 28 when he should logically be ready to die, he begins a "pain cure" to fight death. From an early age, in childhood and adolescence, he had practised hard masochism (entire nights spent naked in the freezing air or up in the air with his wrists tied up, flagellation with a belt studded with nails...) His encounter with a young woman, Sheree, led him, like Dan with Pam, into a sadomasochistic relationship of a particular, quite exhibitionist kind. He made an artistic creation of his torments by performing in art galleries, exhibiting his body in pain like a piece of modern art and also by filming his life with Sheree, particularly their sadomasochistic sessions. I can well believe P. Miller when he says the film is unbearable. *To be sick* means in English to be ill but also to want to vomit. Perhaps more in British English, but the Americans obviously know this meaning too. Bob Flanagan must have been aware of the provocative aspects of his exhibitionism. What we are seeing is megalomaniac narcissism - and Bob considers himself a "supermasochist". Was it this narcissistic demand or his continually increasing need for pain that made him imagine more and more severe tortures, as M. did? Perhaps he also wanted to increase the effectiveness of that strange way of curing illness, by pain.

When we read Miller's work we are profoundly affected. Firstly by the masochistic horrors, discreetly described, almost forcing the author to leave the cinema, and secondly because paradoxically it depicts a world of mothering which Bob Flanagan never knew. The real mother seen in the film appears "harsh, rigid, with an unbelievable murderous violence". However, note the mother's questioning: "Where was I all that time," when the baby was suffering agony, when the adolescent became masochistic? As I said earlier, what stimulus barrier can a mother offer when the violence of a painful and constant stimulus is caused by illness?

And yet Sheree says that what she makes Bob's body endure involves "motherly skills". What is the meaning of the love/hate relationship between Bob and his body? What is the meaning of the one between the two lovers? This very fine work by Miller is essential reading. *It makes me feel invincible. I'm nothing but a big baby.* These two sentences amaze us. Omnipotence of a baby which holds out its hand to the pain of the past by inflicting on itself the pain of today. A baby that triumphs by controlling body, mother and pain. A baby that gives itself the illusion of also controlling the form which the repetitive force took within it, i.e. the constant immovable pain that had to be worked through to control it by replacing passivity with activity fantasies. In both Bob and Dan, the brutal masochistic cathexis drains the essential possibilities massively but not entirely. Both were able to experience a love affair in their own way and both gave themselves up to sublimatory, artistic activity. It was when Bob became more of an artist and gave up his masochistic practices that he died, aged 43. His wager on survival through pain won him 15 years.

I cannot leave the subject of pain desired without briefly mentioning a strong tendency in the modern world to place a higher value on erotic masochism. This is the case above all with the minor sadomasochistic practices (or not) which I have just mentioned when talking about these young women, and which are becoming more popular as a weird kind of fashion statement. The sadomasochistic erotic world seems to be more significant in an age when patients demand hospitals without pain from the medical establishment. A sociologist told me that when an earthquake caused thousands of deaths in a very localised area of Chile, the number of suicides in the country as a whole fell sharply, so that the mortality rate due to accidents and suicides remained at the normal average. Must humanity pay a continuous tribute to death and pain?

A recent book by David Le Breton entitled *Signs of Identity* (2002) reveals some astonishing practices which seem to be spreading fast. His work is subtitled "Tattooing, piercing and other body marks". Pain is the essential condition which underlies all these practices. It may be denied. A certain J.-R. covered his arms and hands with cigarette burns but said that "the pain does not hurt" and if he wanted to cut off his leg he would. These practices are also a way of challenging and provoking society. They are a means of existing against and in opposition and a mark of membership of an underground.

Pain can also be magnified and become an almost mystical experience denied to the uninitiated. The famous fakir Musufar who undergoes amazing tortures in public (such as hanging himself from hooks embedded in his flesh) says of it: "People say that it is incredibly painful, but I say that it is ecstatic and marvellous... the consciousness must be separated". He refers to an orgasm that purifies the orgasm.

What is surprising about Le Breton's book is the commonplace expression of suffering by the people questioned. The role of the object is important, for example the relationship with the tattooist or piercer, both accomplice and tormentor.

Embellishing the body, changing it, perfecting it, fulfilling oneself in the ecstasy of pain, rediscovering primitivism in tattooing (although the original ethnic tradition has been lost), and seeking a personal or group meaning in the marks on the body, all this attests to a search for identity; but the ever-present need to suffer is so strong that here again the mystery of pain keeps its secrets.

Finally, I must mention the terribly painful surgery that Chinese girls undergo when they think they are too small to find a husband or an interesting job. The bones in the leg are broken and connected to an external metal cage containing a device that stretches the leg every day, at the cost of unbearable pain. Sleep is virtually impossible. All this over several months to gain seven or eight centimetres!

A DIFFERENT PAIN CURE

Over a long period my algologist somatic colleagues and I noticed that patients suffering psychogenic pain or pain due to post-traumatic lesions did not have psychosomatic disorders. It was as if they were protected by the pain in a way that was hard to understand. Psychosomaticians for their part wondered why some of their patients had a lack of cathexis vis-à-vis psychic and sometimes physical pain. An attitude that cannot be described as neutral, due to the hysterical model which is certainly not theirs. To caricature them, our patients at the pain clinic are noisy while theirs are silent, at least when they experience the form of suffering which is essential depression. Claude Smadja (1999) wrote a very good and balanced article which clarifies this subject.

In a 1990 article, Jean-Paul Obadia describes an observation which tends to indicate a protective and even curative role of psychosomatic illness. The patient was suffering from rheumatoid arthritis complicated by serious eye lesions: iritis, iridocyclitis and bilateral retinitis which threatened her vision. The patient had been referred to the psychosomatician by her ophthalmologist and agreed to undergo psychotherapy to "play the game". The vivid description given by J.-L. Obadia requires no further comment here. I shall only give the minimal details of the fascinating case he describes that are necessary to pursue my questioning about pain.

Five months after an episode of essential depression containing a touch of melancholia, the patient's arthritis occurred, soon complicated by retinopathy. The psychotherapy proceeded satisfactorily in the sense that the patient both worked through her problems and cathected more and more, even asking to increase the number of sessions. She was much better and her condition stabilised, which meant gradual withdrawal of the steroids and longer intervals between medical checks.

It was then that a sort of perverse invasion occurred which split her in two. She bought lots of sexy underwear, dressed provocatively and took a "gentle and brutal" lover with whom she fulfilled her masochistic desires. Once a week (as with the psychotherapist) she was whipped, beaten and sodomised and she loved it. At the same time, she became closer and much more tender towards her husband.

This masochism/tenderness division is interesting. It may not be a split in the real sense, since it appears more functional than structural. We can see a psychic development in the patient, liberating her from what J.-P. Obadia convincingly calls a "temporary retreat" of the psyche by consideration of the potential for preconscious links and capacity for autoerotic connections in the face of the purely quantitative. This facilitates regression towards essential depression, the operative life and somatic illness. But the evocation of the unconscious sense of guilt, and need for punishment which he invokes to explain the joyful and triumphant emergence of the masochistic erotic process remains enigmatic. It is plausible and it is Freudian. Freud wrote (1919): "Every time the sense of guilt is the factor which changes sadism into masochism". The rapprochement with the husband can be considered as a way of asking for forgiveness or a part of the price to be paid, the other part being the pain received erotically, pleasure, but also punishment. Depending on the case, the enigma lies either in the "temporary retreat" of the psyche which enables the somatic illness to erupt or in the return of the psyche, via the sense of guilt and the triumph of the submission to punishment.

Nevertheless, the enigma remains. The examples of perverse masochism given earlier raise the question of a strong recourse to pain. Although the problems cannot be compared, the recourse to pain of J.-P. Obadia's patient, despite being quantitatively different, perhaps raises the same question, as does the actual title of the article: "When the birth of a masochistic perversion takes over from a serious somatic disorder". The question is that of the function of masochism and its associated pain, a function which appears therapeutic as a result of better economic organisation - the sign of a more complex and flexible psychic reorganisation - now open to potential cathexes as a result of the psychotherapy.

That said, the joyful and even jubilant masochism of this patient bears no relation to that of the great perverse masochists I have discussed. I once had occasion to be present at the emergence of a very similar perverse episode during conventional treatment of a patient. Initially the psychoanalytical structure (four sessions a week) allowed the patient to express the laments of an ego wounded in early life (unknown father, mother whose fragile psyche often broke down in depressive and interpretative episodes) but to contain them. I somehow managed to withstand the violent attacks directed at me. Then the situation improved. At that time various somatic manifestations appeared which seemed to worry her doctors. They increased the blood and body fluid tests (assuming auto-immune disease). "I seem to be destroying myself," she said.

The erotic sadomasochistic episode then erupted, quite moderate in tone but similar to what J.-L. Obadia describes. I was astounded by the affects of exaltation and triumph directed against me that the young woman displayed, in total subjection to the man who had triggered a lateral revenge transference against me. She experienced just as much pleasure in her feelings of *revenge* as in her *submission* to her perverse lover. I have highlighted the words she used. The perverse episode lasted only a few months and ended as suddenly as it had begun, as if it had never existed and had left no trace. Afterwards she could to begin to express a sense of guilt, tentative at first. The analysis resumed its course in a more normal way and genuine, interpretable transference was established. I think my patient had been able to decondense a frightening image of combined parents to allow scope for fantasies of a less sadistic primal scene. This was certainly the function of this perverse episode but does not explain its mechanism. As for the somatic problems, not another word was said about them. Perhaps they had never existed.

These two young women are a reminder of Freud's article quoted above: "A child is being beaten"- a fantasy in three acts, studied by Freud mainly in its female version. The first act is drawn from the memory of a real scene: someone (who will prove to be the father) is beating a hated child, for example a younger brother or sister or someone representing them. It is no coincidence, as M. Fain emphasised, that the adult administering the beating is furious at that moment. The fantasy is sadistic or impregnated with sadism. The second act remains unconscious and can only be a construction of the analysis. It has become masochistic: "I am being beaten by my father." Thus the guilty conscience is appeased. It is the "punishment for the forbidden genital relationship with the father, but also its regressive substitute". It is the source of the libidinal stimulus which will be discharged in masturbation. The third act lives on under the title "A child is being beaten" which retains its stimulating potential and masturbatory discharge. The associated fantasies have a sadistic appearance but enable masochistic satisfaction to be obtained.

In the two young women, the fantasy world is not the secret motor of the erotic fantasy. It overflows. They proclaim it and above all they move to action. They do not dream about the fantasy, which thus loses its function or rather acquires a different one. They want to live it in the reality of the flogging scene, to put themselves in a submissive position and actually suffer the whip. There is a great difference. The stimulus and discharge must pass through the body. As though the psychic stimulus of the evocation of the scene has to lead to the even greater stimulus of the masochism session, which is a genuine acting out of the imaginary scene. I wondered whether this was due to insufficient or, conversely, excessive fantasisation. I believe that both are true. The fantasy world is powerful but locked in its repetitive straitjacket. Would Freud again describe this as genetic?

Without doubt we have to go back to the nature of the first autoerotic activity of these subjects. Obadia thinks that autoeroticism can be considered as a bridge between psyche and soma, "a stuttering of the drive movement in its first defensive processes" (eroticisation of the passivity). He underlines the role of primal erogenous masochism as the first trace of union between soma and psyche, particularly in relation to the pleasing retention of the stimulus. I agree, and believe that primal erogenous masochism plays a fundamental part in the formation of the ego and generates "this new psychic action" - referred to by Freud in his article on narcissism (1914) - which forms its basis when added to autoeroticism. It ensures the repatriation of the drive to what will become the ego. That there is the possibility of physical pain in the vicissitudes of this process is certain. But it cannot be imagined without adding the nature of the anti-cathexis that conditions the original drive repression, the organiser of the future psyche. G. Szwec (1998) stresses the part played by the mother in the process of anti-cathexis, her complicity through her libidinal cathexis of the zones and functions and the drive intricacies that she allows; In short, her work of psychisation. I shall return to this point, processing of the stimulus, in the chapter on treatment.

FUNCTIONS OF FANTASIES AND THEIR NECESSITY

I now want to discuss two points which will be developed later about the roles and functions of pain. The first concerns the fantasy "A child is being beaten".

The main phase of the series of fantasies in Freud's article is the second: "My father is beating me". It is unconscious because it is closest to the secret Oedipal desire. The subject only has a diluted consciousness of it: "A child is being beaten", which is enough to arouse a pleasurable affect and perhaps the move to the act.

In the article, it is the *perception* of a furious adult beating a hated child that is the source of the fantasy, not a *sensation* or the *memory* of a personal sensation. This perception produces a thought, an idea. The memory and evocation of the totally pleasing scene brings repetitive recall and psychic elaboration. The perception and the psychic process based on it bring the subject into this scene which must probably feed on a fantasy of a primal sado-masochistic scene.

We can see here the role of pain in the recall in general and in the elaboration of the fantasy. The two are connected. It is an old idea of Freud's, already contained in "Project for a Scientific Psychology" (p. 347). Lateral facilitations are a diversion from access to the unpleasant memory, and distract the stimulus towards other connected or related memories, which are more pleasant but are connected in some way to the memory avoided. They encircle and accompany this unpleasant or painful memory by means of a network of images with a defensive but representative function. Therefore they retain the stimulus. The psyche can work things through and complexify. The fantasy can be born.

The second indicates once again the protective aspect of pain.

The fantasies of the great perverse masochists are obviously quite different from those of the two young women. The former talk of humiliation, debasement and above all arrogance based on megalomania. In contrast to these violent affects, the others express more muted affects of submission, desire for belonging and pride. Perhaps these are two extremes, heavy to light, of the perverse masochistic world. I am not competent enough to say more. But I still feel that the idea of a struggle against death, the need to keep it at a distance or the pledge of a better life is present. The torments endured, even in the "heavy" category" do not cause death in the examples quoted. "The sadist always chickens out". Although the essence of the masochism and its original expression are the result of fusion of the life and death instincts, the pain desired paradoxically is present throughout life (but is it so paradoxical?). In some subjects it may even be its witness, guarantor and insurance.

Where is the satisfaction? In the actual suffering which causes pleasure and orgasm or in the fantasy? It is hard to say. Probably in both. Freud writes about the economic problem of masochism:

> "The first interpretation discovered without difficulty (!) is that the masochist wants to be treated like a *small child* in *distress and dependent* but he *wants* above all to be treated like a *naughty child*." (Freud, 1924)

I have always found this quotation mysterious and I have italicised the most surprising points. It invokes the origins: infancy, dependence and distress, and the desire: the child *wants*. But why should naughtiness and pleasure be linked? Is the purpose the punishment that goes with it or a primal desire for cruelty or destruction? There may be a chain involved: Naughtiness, parent or another, furious, punishment. In the article "A child is being beaten", flogging is the primary idea and it is only later that we have the idea of being punished and humiliated, in the cases where the fantasy is conscious due to a clever superstructure of awakened dreams. These cultivated fantasies of submission, humiliation or even enslavement and the affects of arrogance and pride associated with them denote the importance of the narcissistic reinforcement sought and obtained.

In the same article Freud tells us that the expression of the need for punishment can be replaced by the "psychologically incorrect" one of an unconscious sense of guilt. Certainly, it is difficult for us to imagine unconscious affects or feelings. They appeared in The Ego and the Id (1923) and Freud explains them without giving a clear idea of what is involved, except that it evokes the "tensions of the needs" of the "driving forces" of the Id. They act without the ego perceiving the compulsion it is undergoing. Freud even alludes to an unconscious pain which is due to a need. There is a need to suffer which is close to the need for punishment without being part of it. This is a different explanation for masochism, making it not only an ability to bear tension and pain, allowing life, but more of a desire and a need to suffer. It is this latter need, attributed to a true reversal of the instinct for self-preservation, that Freud (in the basic writings, 1938) gives as the reason for one of the two variants of resistance to psychoanalysis, the other being the need to be ill. But it this a reason? Why the hurt? asks A. Green in *Private Madness* (1990): He is tempted to paraphrase the words of Angelus Silesius: "The rose exists without a reason".

Hurt too?

Part 3

Theory and Treatment

Chapter 8

MELANCHOLIA OF THE BODY: ALGOSIS OR ALGETIC NEUROSIS

> *"But the ego can only draw the same conclusion when it finds itself in a real and excessive danger which it does not feel able to overcome by its own efforts. It sees itself abandoned by all the protective powers and allows itself to die. It is the same situation that was at the heart of the first great anxiety state, birth, and of the infantile nostalgia anxiety, separation from the protective mother."*
>
> *Freud,* The Ego and the Id, *p. 274*

Two main themes are interwoven in this third part: the first part is theoretical and is an examination and elaboration of the reasons for the presence, intensity and above all permanence of chronic physical pain once it has appeared; the second part is more clinical and raises questions about the methods of treating it psychically, i.e. establishing a therapeutic relationship with chronic pain patients so that they can either manage it better or be free of it.

Pain raises theoretical questions. It seems normal to us that it should be an invasion felt to be "unpleasant", as its international definition indicates (Merskey 1979), because all pain felt by humans is immediately cathected and even hypercathected. It breaks through the normal boundaries. It is not cathected by psychic choice but because one cannot escape doing so. This hypercathexis necessitated by the acute, sudden or intense nature of the pain normally diminishes gradually, but it remains present and above all continuous if the cause of the pain persists.

If it becomes chronically established, various alternatives can be envisaged. The clinical aspect of chronic pain sufferers is very heterogeneous and polymorphic. Two extremes mark their limits:

- The first consists of disorders such as hypochondria or some post-traumatic pathologies which are painful and unleash intense complaints, although they are only accompanied by minimal or non-existent somatic lesions. The patients are called psychogenic because pain has to have a cause.
- The second is perhaps even more enigmatic: the disorders called psychosomatic in which complaints of pain are not heard even though they are due to lesions which are sometimes serious, sometimes mortal and often hyperalgesic. The patients are then called alexithymic, unexpressive of their suffering.

Therefore pain does not imply complaint and complaint does not imply a lesion. It is complaint that leads our patients to consult us.

Does this mystery raise the question of a possible protective function of pain against somatisation, a lesional attack on the body lesion? This question is increasingly being asked by our psychosomatician colleagues. It is no doubt up to us, the algologists, to try to answer it. Later on I shall try to shed some light on this difficult and enigmatic aspect which is valuable because it clarifies the problem of pain.

At all events, these two opposite groups define the extremes of the world of pain that is complex but united by characteristics common to all patients who complain of it.

In this chapter I shall show how the pain clinic supplied fuel for the theory and how, in return the theory supplied knowledge for the clinical practice that developed in time.

A HEALTHY BODY IS ALSO THE MOTHER'S CONSTRUCTION

Original pain, the pain in the distress of the newborn (Freud's *Hilflosigkeit*), the pain associated with its impotence, and the vanity of the ascendancy instinct which is an extension of it, is a fact of life.

Therefore a body without pain is something acquired. The mother's role is to take away pain from a body suffering at that instant. This is the place and role of consolation. Pain can be felt by a baby outside painful stimuli because it has a function of appeal to the consoling mother. This is the stimulus barrier function assigned to her.

Therefore the idea is that a healthy, pain-free body, which on some level is taken for granted, has also to be a construction of the mother. An appeal repeatedly unheard ends by hurting the child. Its normal cenaeshesia, which goes from pain to well being, is formed within the affective relationship. If this is good, the change from laughter to tears will not seriously affect it. It will have confidence in the parental presence. It can voice its affects and can exchange.

If not, it will get into the habit of expressing itself (in addition to language) through physical affects which I call primal, into the body: crying, pain, agitation, rage, anger etc. Overused facilitations leave engrams and provide an easy route to behavioural and emotional responses when the circumstances are right. I am convinced that the lumbar location of certain algia that follow minor accidents accompanied by few lesions or none at all is linked to traumatic circumstances such as abandonment, or a sudden change in the affective environment that occurred at an age when the baby was learning to control its spinal column (sitting and standing) between six months and a year old.

In the baby, the appropriation of the body is accompanied by the history of its ceneasthetic sensations, which all leave traces and are associated with the after-images of the subject's desires, frustrations and wounds. This is the body's affective memory. The subject's past will shape its world of experience of pain. Some foods begin to be liked and others hated. The same applies to pain. The body remembers. Pain is categorised in this way in the course of time and triggers unpredictable behaviours, fears and even pusillanimity. What we are looking at here is masochism and its ability to retain the excitation quantitatively and to retain the discharge.

But there is also a qualitative aspect. One painful sensation will be tolerated while another of similar intensity will cause intense suffering. We know people who can only bear to have injections in one part of the body, right or left, and others who are afraid of eye pain but not toothache, etc. There are some who hate vomiting and others who find relief in it. When treating pain sufferers, it is important to take note of these peculiarities when they are expressed because they lead to recollections, often very old, and valuable associations.

The body modelled by the mother has to be recaptured and reappropriated by working through rejection and separation from her. "One body for two" wrote Joyce McDougall. The baby must construct and appropriate its own corporality, a body of its own. In other words the world of its anatomy and physiology. Accepting them requires effort. We know that this effort is challenged at puberty. A nose which was no problem becomes shiny or misshapen, a back is too bent, the arms are too long or too short. Adolescence can easily become dysmorphophobic.

After the reappropriation, if the internal objects are built on good-quality narcissistic foundations – a sign that the mother has dreamed of the baby and it has been able to dream of her – the subject acquires consolability, as American authors call it, and above all the capability for self-consolation deriving from it, that is the capacity for self-reparation. This is not always the case.

If pain is the result of constructions and deconstructions within the structure of the relationship with the mother, there should be optimism about the possibility of treating it. In a maternal, consoling position, the analyst should be able to relieve his patient's pain. Not so: the chronic pain sufferer, or at least the type that frequents pain clinics, is inconsolable. What can we offer him? And why is it so difficult?

Before considering the options for psychotherapy of pain drawn from experience, I must introduce the obdurate adversary we have to face.

PAIN AS A BLACK HOLE: ALGOSIS

> "The melancholic complex behaves like an open wound attracting cathexis energies (those which we called anti-cathexis in transference neuroses) to it from all sides and draining the ego until it completely impoverishes it." (Freud, 1917)

This quotation from *Mourning and Melancholia* is perfectly apt for the situation of established chronic pain. The pain is a black hole attracting all the cathexis energies and causing narcissistic overtension (J. Cournut). The external objects are lost in this cathexis emptiness and if they had performed a function of external support due to the failings of poor-quality internal objects, the whole ego is wrecked. Freud told us that the lost objects or new substitute objects can only be recathected by distraction, i.e. by rerouting some of the energy immobilised by the black hole and redistributing it. This is difficult work because of the algosis, the genuine physical melancholia which rebels against any attempt at detachment from the pain substance.

I want to advance a theory which does not divide chronic pain into nosographic categories but tries to understand it differently: That algosis or "algetic neurosis" consists of firstly cathecting an existing pain, a painful feeling or simply a cenaesthesia by perceiving or associating with it a certain level of pain intensity, and secondly surrendering to real cultivation of the pain phenomenon. The first stage meets a basic human need shared by us all. The second is more complex and involves the subject's psychic organisation.

This is a general predisposition in human beings because pain is subjective, but some subjects have a particular capacity for feeling and cultivating pain. Cathexis of pain is one thing but cultivation is quite another. It is linked to a powerful masochistic renewal of the first cathexis. This defensive cathexis of pain stems from the psyche and curiously bypasses it, which is often the object of the exercise. It is in the intensity of feeling and its continuous maintenance that pain - in the form of algetic neurosis or algosis - can be used as a psychic solution of pain. It is often preferred to anxiety or any other psychic symptom because it is seen as more robust and reliable and less dangerous because it avoids intrapsychic conflict. Anxiety retains very close links with the things that motivate it. It can be their signal. Physical pain, locked in its own intensity, has the security of the body to ignore a possible internal conflict.

Algetic neurosis has nothing to do with pusillanimity or softness. It originates from the human capacity to cathect pain, preserve it and even produce it forcefully, whether or not there is a somatic lesion.

This capacity appears very regressive. It corresponds to a very archaic and early psychic position which prefers a physical to a psychic symptom, and dates back to a period when somatic and psychic were more or less merged. It means that subjects rediscover a strongly marked point of certainty from their past. The solution of pain represents its possibility; algosis or algetic neurosis represents the result, when pain has become established as a solution. Sensation is preferred to affect, which risks reviving the psyche and what has been repressed. Therefore it is a defence.

It helps to combat the return of distress once experienced. We have seen that this is the case with lumbalgics and hypochondriacs, but it applies to many others who consult us as well. Physical pain is a paradoxical defensive recourse – a delayed after-shock from early disasters and what are sometimes called "emptiness neuroses". Once cathected, it can become a psychic symptom similar to anxiety or anything else (phobias, obsessions, behavioural problems etc.); a recourse and therefore a solution.

It is not restricted to hypochondriacs, psychogenic lumbalgics and hysterics. Every pain sufferer presents with a period of algosis to a greater or lesser degree. As we have seen, hypochondriacs have gone through it instantly and therefore very early and partialised, in the sense that they have sacrificed a painful part to save the whole. They have somehow cut their psychic space in two, whereas lumbalgics have gone through it in two stages, first heaven then hell. In their case the breach has occurred over time.

Back pain sufferers are the best example because the causal lesion is minimal or non-existent and yet their pain feels very intense and above all incurable and permanent. Psychosomatic patients are the opposite, they have lesions which are sometimes very painful and may be serious (arthritis or rectocolitis) but complain little or not at all and pose no particular problems to somaticians as far as pain is concerned.

I think that algosis exists to a very high degree in the former (psychogenics) and is very weak, non-existent or even negative in the latter (who have still somatised). It can therefore be measured by the complaints. Between these two extremes there is an average algosis representing a relatively neutral way of perceiving the physiological signal of pain, i.e. with the minimum of translation. This is the most frequent case. Fortunately, no-one has invented a machine to measure pain and estimate whether its intensity is justifiable when set against the algogenic potential of the causal lesion.

If patients suffer and complain, it is because they have reason to do so and these reasons interest the psychoanalyst and the humanist in him. There is an immense and fascinating field here which has been neglected by analysts, whereas the non-existent or minimal complaints of psychosomatic patients - which were an even greater mystery to me than the noisy complaints of the psychogenics - have attracted the attention of our psychosomatician colleagues.

Curiously, there is a "pharmacological" translation of this distinction between the two categories. Analgesics, with morphine if necessary, are effective in treating the pain of psychosomatic patients, in which case patients and doctors are, so to speak, satisfied. Lumbalgics, unresponsive to all pharmacopoeia, are not at all satisfied. They can continue their complaints to their therapists, who are just as unsatisfied. Once again, I am speaking of the lumbalgics called psychogenic; those in pain due to major lesions are eminently treatable. It is the psychogenic patients who will explain the conditions under which pain becomes established as a solution and perhaps ask a relevant question to be discussed later: does the pain, or the hyperactivity which can precede it, guard against a psychosomatic affliction?

The pattern of melancholia in which the ego is crushed under the weight of its sense of guilt therefore has its response in the pattern of algosis in which the physical pain and the complaints it provokes, replaces the mental pain and the guilt. Like the melancholic complaints, algosis also occurs after a loss or what is perceived as a loss. The physical pain, frequently the primary cause of the loss, often becomes the reason that makes the loss irrecoverable. Why do lumbalgics, those workaholics, stop all activity after their accident? Because they are suffering. In other cases, physical suffering which somaticians find mysterious takes the place of a different kind of suffering, the mental suffering of mourning now avoided.

The algosis symptom which claims to be outside the psyche seeks to hide from any psychic effort. The body instead of the mind. And yet the algosis, which *retains* the physical pain, is firmly rooted in the psyche. It is that part of the psyche which clings to an opportunistic pain of physiological origin (or creates it if necessary), and self-maintains and self-aggravates it by assigning a basic defensive function to it, and profoundly reorganising the ego.

ANTI-CATHEXIS

What psychoanalytical defence can we think of? On the subject of energetic anti-cathexis, a sort of dynamic parapet neutralising the violence of the invasion, I feel that Freud's 1920 metaphor should not be taken too far, except to utilise it in its true meaning. My first point will be unification rather than separation of the combatants. The two forces present in this situation – the trauma of the pain and the counter-force which tries to suppress it – are actually one and the same. It is impossible to distinguish the two adversaries in the melee. The confusion which the combat might represent is the subject of a single cathexis which merges attacker and defender, and can only be understood with the complicity of masochism. The important point is the indisputable impoverishment of the ego and its inability to re-enrich itself. The clinic shows us on a daily basis the picture that Freud described so well in *Beyond the Pleasure Principle*. But perhaps this is the first phase and we do not have to share his pessimism? When Freud talks of pain, he does not distinguish it from the complaints it generates, "ineradicable in ø", as if it were obvious. Psychosomatic patients show that this is not an absolute rule. It is the complaint or need for complaint of some patients which poses the problem of pain. It has left us with a pattern of defence with an immutable, powerful, autofunctional and sometimes self-aggravating anti-cathexis. This is actually found in cases where the complaint is incurable, with no outcome on offer other than distraction, to redistribute the energy absorbed by the pain to old cathexes or new ones replacing them, a centrifugal force to achieve freedom from the attraction of pain.

Pain has an antipsychic effect, like trauma which is closely linked to it. Whether the psyche is struck dumb as in trauma or impoverished as in pain, it is wounded and incapable of performing its normal functions.

But it is time to leave this purely energetic standpoint and examine what happens qualitatively. To be precise, the reorganisation of the ego when it becomes wholly painful and the various changes which are necessary for it to defend itself, survive and adapt. There is no doubt that this hypercathexis of the pain gives it substance and intensifies it. A different integration of the painful psychic experience first involves decathexis of the "hyper" aspect. This can occur spontaneously.

Two alternatives need to be considered:

- In the first one, when the pain invades the ego, the person affected hypercathects the pain, which is normal. But if the object and narcissistic cathexes (affective, family, professional, leisure etc.) that structure and organise the life of the psyche are robust, what will happen sooner or later is a means of refusing cathexis of the pain and reflux of the energy absorbed by it to abandoned cathexes, in order to re-establish them. Once again this presupposes robust and reliable internal objects. They will then form a sort of pain barrier. This is the most frequent case: "Pain or not, I have to go ...", this subject says where possible, while the pain sufferer fixed in algosis thinks: "I cannot go ... because I am in too much pain". In this case the attraction exerted by the structural cathexes is stronger than that exerted by the pain, while the opposite is true in the other case. These cathexes offer a channel to reroute the energy immobilised by the pain and become an object of distraction which alone is capable of soothing pain, according to Freud. I repeat that algetic neurosis has nothing to do with being soft; no-one is tougher than a lumbalgic... until the accident. But once the pain has established itself, the objects previously cathected become inaccessible and it is unthinkable to find new ones, which is the purpose of the therapy.

- In the second case therefore, the pain is also strongly cathected, for reasons that have to do with the subject's past. But it is not cathected against, it is cathected for. More precisely, as I shown earlier, pain and its anti-cathexis form one solid, unshakeable entity which has found its raison d'être. This is the black hole. In lumbalgics and many other patients too, it replaces the hyperactivity which was itself a defence, with one difference: it is infinitely more firmly rooted. I shall come back to the back pain patients because they give us a chance to understand the reason for the process and its mechanism.

Between these two alternatives there are intermediate positions in which some subjects cultivate a small painful world, often much cathected for narcissistic reasons, or the memory of past distress, a small secret enclave which varies in size but does not prevent them living their lives. This applies to many of our "cured" patients.

Lumbalgics progress from hypercathexis of activity to hypercathexis of pain. The loss object is therefore disproportionate. Its disappearance leads to considerable reorganisation of the ego which shall be described in detail in the clinical section. It is the model, in schematic and greatly magnified form, of what occurs in all chronic pain sufferers.

HYPERACTIVITY AND PAIN

The life history of a lumbalgic can be broken down as follows:

1. Original distress
2. Hyperactivity
3. Accident ending all activity
4. Pain

And it is what can also be observed in many chronic pain sufferers, including minor post-traumatic patients, with the different points acquiring varying degrees of importance. We have to try to understand this sequence in its chronological order. Hyperactivity, which anti-cathects the original distress, does not impoverish the ego in back pain sufferers. Quite the reverse, it shapes and enriches it constantly, even if the ego is externalised. The continuously repeated outward diversion of the drive excitations represents a more reliable object than the internal one. It is reliable but fragile and maintains its weakness precisely from the lack of reliability of the internal strata. Because the internal object is unreassuring, it forces the lumbalgic to create a reliable external object outside, like an external spinal column or carapace. This is not the case with the psychosomatic patient, or less so.

Therefore the hyperactivity was itself an anti-cathexis of the distress, effective but requiring the patient to keep running to avoid falling. If any incident interrupts it and pain follows, it is replaced by a different anti-cathexis, the one that Freud spoke of when discussing pain (in *Beyond the Pleasure Principle*).

Hyperactivity has many functions. It has enabled the patient to replace the deficient object. The object was previously missing but is now lost. Hyperactivity has an anti-traumatic role which is later replaced paradoxically by pain. By cathecting outwards, the back pain sufferer decathects the deficient internal object and finally adopts an active attitude. The process can be seen like this: in moments "of instant pressures" associated, for example, with feelings of abandonment or rejection, the baby cannot construct a consoling mother internally and looks outside. It escapes from its mother and out of her line of fire but things are unfinished and it is a bad beginning.

In short, it is the game of the bobbin diverted from its goal and cathected for itself and not to master the game of the mother's absences by alternate appearances and disappearances. This was what Freud's grandson did by pulling the thread or throwing out the bobbin, enabling him to create an internal space capable of containing the stimuli. He could think of his mother.

The future lumbalgic thinks outwardly. His game becomes creative, clever and adaptable. Unlike what is said about the operant patient who cathects the factual as and when he needs to, he invents, controls and constructs in an atmosphere of joy and contentment. He tries to repair his mother by repairing the world: the stimulus has found its discharge and the patient has found a means of control.

But he does much more. He reunifies and renarcissises his ego through the satisfaction he experiences, preserving his self-esteem; in short he is a mother to himself and also to others. I have always been impressed by the devotion and desire to care for others of these previously hyperactive patients. Also, because the activity is linked to the perception of the motor function, its cathexis and the resultant success generate a feeling of triumph which further reinforces the ego, due to all the secondary benefits obtained (gratitude from others, reputation and recognition). In contrast, the pain is experienced as a defeat.

All this gives birth to a feeling of self-begetting which is not wholly unjustified. The subject may legitimately think that he only owes his origins to himself. The problem is that there is no room for negation in his system. Affirmation, continually repeated, reigns supreme. There is no apparent conflict. The object is more than incidental; it is vague, diverse and constantly replaced by a different one, in a game repeated by necessity. The problem of repetition is initiated. All repetition is doubtless an attempt at imagination, but in the world of hyperactivity and of the pain that follows it, the repetition loses this status. It is merged and dissolved into a world that will never allow it to fulfil its imaginative destiny.

Above all, this resolutely activity-based position is a dynamic anti-cathexis against the destructive drive towards the mother and the hatred once felt. The muscular and motor functions have found the object elsewhere, on the outside, but at the cost of unending movement. The situation appears fragile, but in an age when stress has replaced psychic problems, our modern world is full of people who keep on running and never fall.

This is not the case with lumbalgics, some of whom will experience what they most fear, the end of their activity. The fact that an accident – sometimes trivial - is the reason why they stop shows their unfitness and refusal to tolerate inactivity. It is this refusal that drives them to accept everything that life has to offer, and enables them to practise the skills acquired as a result of their liking for activity. They always have something to do.

The basic essentials are not there: all the psychic neo-organisation, giving them effective protection against an internal mother kept at a distance, means a psyche which must maintain that distance constantly. Reunions with the hated object are impossible. But when the pain replaces the hyperactivity which can be said to be its symmetrical opposite, the old phantoms can resurface. Then the pain takes over the defensive role through its incurability. The patient has replaced the thanks he received from others by the complaints he directs towards them.

We can see the similarity between the two defences. They have the same function: to prevent the distress returning. Constant stimulus is maintained in both cases. Through the pain, but also through the hyperactivity, stimuli and discharges are merged and self-maintained. Both autoeroticisms - painful and hyperactive - reinforce the narcissism, each in its own way. They also enable the aggression to be denied or turned onto others. The complaints of pain expressed, the demands for help and the passivity which are characteristic of chronic pain represent a tyranny which is a way of exerting control; it is the omnipotence of passivity.

The hyperactivity has to be seen in the context of the relationship with the mother. In these cases, hyperactivity can constitute a defence against the excessive or inadequate (but unmanageable) stimuli of maternal origin. The mother is decathected without being destroyed and the hyperactivity replaces her. The object is now outside. What happens to the internal object? A hole, a void. It is effaced. The continuous cathexis avoids reviving the dead mother and her place is taken. The mother is repressed. The cathexis of external reality is a cathexis against the mother, who vanishes and is therefore a defensive anti-cathexis. The bobbin had no thread.

In both cases the body has been used, either as an agent of the hyperactivity or in an apparently passive way in the pain. I say apparently because the amount of energy used in the hyperactivity and its reversal into pain removes much of the meaning from the word passive. The problem is not in the passivity, it is in the reversal. The externalised aggression has returned to its starting point, pain, but does not know it.

This dynamic anti-cathexis which harnesses the available energy impoverishes the ego by forcing a repetitive, indigent function on it. But it draws solidity from it and appears firm and unshakeable. The lumbalgic gives us an opportunity to see what its peculiarities are and to have some idea of what therapeutic work might help to break it down: To redistribute the energy mobilised by the anti-cathexis to the "impoverished" regions.

VIBRANCY OF THE PAIN AND MORTIFICATION OF THE STIMULUS BARRIER

I was explaining to an analyst friend one day the two phases that occur in some patients, particularly lumbalgics (i.e. hyperactivity that changes to pain after an accident or incident that is usually minor) and said to him without too much consideration of these rather enigmatic words: "they have preferred the vibrancy of the pain to the mortification of the stimulus barrier". I added that this might explain the difference between the pain sufferers who complain with little reason and the patients called psychosomatic who have lesions but little or no complaint.

Once again we have to go back to the origins, that is to the processing of the excessively early stimuli, and how the mother did or did not soothe and treat them properly. The immature psyche cannot contain or absorb them. The anti-cathexis offered by the mother which should have secured the quality of the original repression did not fulfil this function and left the baby destitute and fragile. What I call the primary affects: rage, anger, distress, anxiety and therefore pain, were not given a meaning and did not nourish the psyche due to a lack of maternal rapport. Using Bion's words, we could say that too many beta elements were not given the transformation to alpha that they could and should have had.

Psychosomaticians who are very interested in this question contemplate psychosomatic responses to the excess of stimuli. C. Smadja (1999) thinks this could involve behaviour which defies psychic classification although the affect starts it. G. Szwec (1996) speaks of a self-calming subversion in place of the normal erotic subversion.

I think that in some infants (future psychosomatic patients) over-stimulus has prevented development of the normal constituent defences of the psyche, but nor have they used the defences of lumbalgics, who have somehow been able to flee the mother and transpose the object outwards to make it controllable. For some reason, these infants have been unable to manufacture effective defences against a caustic mother. They may have identified with the hole and the void, and been locked in poorly elaborated mourning for an object missing, rather than lost and remaining vague. They have taken the full force of the unmanageable stimuli. They have not been able to invent the bobbin game and have preferred the shield of the stimulus barrier, despite the lack of effectiveness of what the mother could offer. The Freudian stimulus barrier should certainly be seen as a metaphor. It does not prevent Freud (in *Beyond the Pleasure Principle*) imagining a stimulus receptor cortical layer on the living vesicle in which the "uppermost layer relinquishes the structure peculiar to the living" and becomes inorganic. This is the mortification I refer to, now a shield. To continue the metaphor, in them everything happens as if the part that has lost its living quality has become porous, ineffective and coarsened. The mortified part has won over the interior, creating space for possible future somatisation. I think that a child like this that takes the full force of the stimuli becomes itself largely a mortified stimulus barrier; to the detriment of the "vibrancy" implied by hyperactivity, another stimulus which is possibly convertible, e.g. to plaintive pain, as with the back pain sufferers.

M. Fain (1992) asks the question in these terms:

> "Can one describe a relationship between two beings during which one is purely a cultivation of the death instinct for the other? An object forcing the subject to deobjectalize (A. Green)?"

He quotes the example of an insomniac baby that cannot fall asleep unless rocked for some time. It cannot experience a hallucination of desire and "without hallucination of the object, primary deobjectalization is established", he adds. The appearance of self-destructive gestures can sometimes be observed in these infants, such as head banging, which can be interpreted as internalisation of the rocking required for sleep. This is no doubt a behaviour pattern *and* a self-calming practice.

G. Szwec (1998) picks up from L. Kreisler the "infantile empty behaviour syndrome" characterised by recourse to behaviour patterns to fill the fantasy void. He refers to the baby's nonobjectal depression and mother avoidance behaviour and to a lack of tokens of affection which make it "unaffectionate". This is all to promote a "psychic disengagement from the relationship". L. Kreisler considers that underlying this syndrome is a "blank depression" caused by a breakdown of the libidinal energy (a preliminary form of essential depression) which leads to deobjectalization, or even non-objectalization, adds G. Szwec.

I think that a phobic reaction of this kind towards the mother really can lead to the position described by L. Kreisler and G. Szwec. But it is not the only one, because the way is then open to two different destinies: The fate of lumbalgics starts from a contraphobic attitude of denial of the anxiety and distress and a plunge into activity, in which the excitation finds satisfaction if the power instinct has room to manoeuvre. In contrast the fate of psychosomatics is a much more passive cultivation of more or less self-calming systems. Calming the drive stimulus is not the same as satisfying it, and the development of the psyche is bound to be seriously affected.

One question arises, that of the detachment from the mother. The process of separation-individuation appears successful in the lumbalgic, but his weak internal structure exposes him to possible fragility and a traumatophilic disposition. He has used the hyperactivity to construct an auxiliary stimulus barrier to compensate for the mother's faulty one. When the pain emerges and invades him, it forms another paradoxical stimulus barrier: He cannot get better, he thinks, but nor can he get worse! He is protected. His destiny is one of life, as shown by his happiness when he is hyperactive, but also by the intensity and appeal of his lamentation when the pain catches up with him.

In my general practice days, I had occasion to meet "unaffectionate" children, as L. Kreisler and G. Szwec describe them. I think this is what A. Ferro (1997) calls "lethargisation", an archaic defence mechanism that consists of putting "the aggression, entire regions of the psyche and often all creative potential" to sleep. But I think it is not so much sleep, as indicated by the word lethargisation, as destructiveness as expressed by the word mortification. Or rather that this sleep - a lack of psychic vitality as a result of repeated attacks which have not been sufficiently discharged - is a defence mechanism like the self-calming solution. But what about the drive discharge, fantasy, self-consolation? Minimum vibrancy. Maximum mortification. This chimes well with the description that psychosomatician analysts give of their patients: Poor fantasy life, few dreams, thinking becoming operant and essential depression, "without an object", in case of difficulty and above all somatic fragility with alexithymia. As the main subject of this book is complaint of pain, I only mention their problems to contrast them with those of our pain sufferers.

Since the idea is that the psyche has not developed as it could have done and if the mind protects the body, as Marty's theory indicates, it is also understandable that this function cannot be fulfilled. It is also understandable that in some cases the stimulus will directly affect the body, without initiating the working through in the psyche that it could have produced.

Therefore there is no possibility for these patients of algosis, i.e. discharge in masochistically cultivated pain. Both pain and hyperactivity have vibrancy (a word that I prefer to vitality because it describes the thing developing – the blossoming), the pain because it gives a feeling of existing and the hyperactivity when it is constructive.

This algosis has several functions:

- To be a paradoxical stimulus barrier;
- To provide a narcissistic position;
- To protect the psyche from elaboration or effort that would bring back the old demons and lead to reunions with the hated object, and often distress;
- To absorb the sense of guilt even more effectively than the hyperactivity did;
- To accuse, through the doctor who is powerless to heal and console, the maternal object who once also failed;
- And, perhaps, to protect against a somatic lesion attack.

DETACHMENT, REVERSAL AND DISTRACTION

A fairly old article by J. Gammil (1989) discussed the case of British pilots who were heroes in fighters or bombers during the Second World War, i.e. in very dangerous situations, but in peacetime were incapable of piloting aircraft which were safe and easy to fly, despite considerable financial inducements. They had become phobic. J. Gammil saw it as the disappearance of a previous contraphobic attitude which had forced them into action and the desire to fly. I was struck by their resemblance to some chronic pain sufferers who are nostalgic for their past activity but are now reduced to inaction. They too had suddenly become incapable, as if they had suddenly felt small and reduced to infancy in a world too big for them. This gave me the idea that their detachment and distraction from a caustic mother could be a phobic reaction, motivated no doubt by the lack of support provided by that mother, but associated with a desire for avoidance, hence their commitment to hyperactivity, contraphobic of external reality.

From this idea came two questions: Why does this behaviour suddenly stop? Why the pain? We could also ask: Why the original contraphobia? The phobic aspect underlined by G. Szwec in the case of the unaffectionate babies is easy to understand. But it is also easy to understand the phobic displacement to another object or the creation of a contraphobic cathexis, for example to any kind of activity, as is the case with many hyperactive subjects.

I would count as one means of distraction the contraphobic commitment that requires something more, rejection of the phobia and a desire to cathect elsewhere. The first phase – phobic – is then a kind of reflex response and the second contraphobic phase is intentional in the wider sense – a psychic necessity. Distraction is the ability to look elsewhere, be interested and cathect, which the future psychosomatic apparently cannot do, and the lumbalgic cannot do again after the accident that plunges him into pain. I use the word distraction because it is the only psychic process that Freud can imagine to turn him away from his pain, the only one capable of combating the attractive force that reversal involves, called by J. Laplanche (1970) the retracing of the drive to the ego when the pain invades.

In his article Gammil is insistent that the child must mourn for the mother in these cases. I think it is more a case of mourning lacking, avoided and left in the air, so that a debt is contracted which has to be paid some day and creates the potential for traumatophilia. Traumatophilia or not, it is inevitable that these things will come back some day. The drive repatriates to the ego. Like any other loss, the loss of hyperactivity or the ability to control is impossible to accept. The mourning cannot be elaborated, cannot be achieved and is transformed into pain which can be physical, a melancholia of the body. We shall take up this point a little later on the subject of the functions of pain.

This phenomenon of reversal of the libido withdrawn from the objects is a recurrent theme in Freud. He mentions it in the work on "Narcissism" (1914), in "Instincts and their Vicissitudes" (1915), *Mourning and Melancholia* (1917), "A child is being beaten" (1919) – where it is used to satisfy a masochistic sexual fantasy – in *Beyond the Pleasure Principle* (1920) and in 1924 in "The economic problem of masochism".

Whether it is a cause, as in masochism in 1924, or a consequence, as in *Instincts*, the theme of pain is almost always central. This may be due to the power of binding that masochism has and its close connection with narcissism, itself a powerful binding and attraction factor. I shall discuss this point again later when comparing regression and reversal.

In the case of chronic pain, the process initiated is not due to the retracing of the drive triggered by an internal causality. The cause is external, foreign to the psyche. It is traumatic. It is not, or not directly, a vicissitude, but the world of the instincts is plunged into masochism.

This is the heart of the enigma of the cathexis of pain in human beings and its processes. The enigma is not one of pain but of masochism, which makes man capable of extending pleasure to pain. Freud said in *Instincts and their Vicissitudes*:

> "But once the transformation into masochism is accomplished, the pains are ideally suited to achieve a passive masochistic aim. We have every reason to accept that sensations of pain, like other sensations of displeasure, overflow into the region of sexual arousal

> and cause a pleasurable state; this is why it is possible to consent to the displeasure of pain." (Freud, 1915)

At that period he thought masochism was a "transformation" of sadism, precisely by reversal; by 1924 it had become inherent and primal.

But what does "...once the transformation into masochism is accomplished," mean? Where does the transformation come from? Is it a fact of Freudian pansexualism or does it involve the mute destitution of the death instinct? Finally, what is the black hole, first and last, the inherent attractive force which drives the pain into the ego?

When the pain is established, it also generates narcissistic overtension which turns the drive cathexes back to the ego, or rather attracts the energy of these cathexes to itself, at the heart of an overwhelmed ego. Despite what stoics say, it is difficult to disregard persistent pain. If this is not the case and it disappears, we can see that the normal cathexes resume of their own accord. But is the opposite true? Does enabling a patient to recathect his objects as he did before the pain dissipate it? This is what psychotherapy for chronic pain sufferers attempts to achieve. I would not have continued to pursue it for more than twenty years if it had been impossible. It is true that only masochism makes the non-occurrence of the reflux of the drive energy to previous cathexes intelligible. So the pain is preserved.

How does it work? Is it, like the image of the double, a token of life or a portent of death? Pain sufferers drift between two suspect, indecisive worlds that evade the question. But the question exists. They experience a reversal which is on the side of the forces of masochism. How can a turning away, drift or distraction that asserts life forces be possible? Who makes us cathect pain or conversely helps us to be free of it? We shall see later in the treatment section that although the process of lateral cathexis (or connected cathexis as Freud calls it) often indicated by patients themselves is not always easy to initiate, it opens up means of disengagement.

I think about all the pain sufferers who come and ask us to relieve their pain and about those who do not come to see us but suffer in silence and ask for nothing. I tell myself that the only difference between them is the necessity, the need for complaint. And that stoicism is not the issue, all that counts is the engrams left within them by their relationship with the primary object and its fate. This brings us back to the question of inherent distress and the beginnings of life.

For Freud there are two origins of pain.

- The first is the initial *Hilflosigkeit*, the primal helplessness which can only be experienced passively and contains an appeal for help.
- The other involves a much more active potential. It is *Bemächtigung*, the drive or need for ascendancy, but also the desire for power urging on the motor functions of the disarmed baby which are unsure and necessarily doomed to defeat.

Primary failure and different appeal for help. There are two roots to human pain, one close to sensation and the body and the other to the newborn feeling of impotence. Castration.

To return to the obscure reason which gives a slight accident, or trivial circumstance the power to precipitate happy, active people who are gratified by the control given them by the motor functions which they have cathected so strongly into passivity and pain. The need for ascendancy - almost megalomaniac in some cases but essential in every way in hyperactive subjects - makes the actual loss, and above all the imaginary loss of that ascendancy, a catastrophe. I am not really sure why hyperactives who have managed to turn away from their distress and pain, and to embrace the world with open arms, are re-embraced by pain and unable to extricate themselves as they did the first time.

In his work on guilt feelings, A. Beetschen (2003) considers the disappointment born of the continual dissatisfaction of the instincts, not just that caused by the lack of ascendancy and the "hostility" that accompanies it. An inherent sense of guilt is the result.

DOES PHYSICAL PAIN PROTECT AGAINST A SOMATIC LESION?

To word the question more precisely, we have to ask whether the physical pain is a warning and activation of an antisomatic protective system within the psyche. This function is defective in the patients called psychosomatic. We find that the chronic pain sufferers who frequent our clinics somatise very little. It is only one step from this to the theory that pain has an antisomatisation effect.

But many of our patients in pain do have somatic lesions. There are two categories: either accidental, post-traumatic or post-surgical, or those based on established disorders (diabetes, cardiovascular disorders, neuralgia etc.) for which our psychosomatician colleagues have no hesitation in asserting the involvement in the aetiology of a process of "psychosomatisation", which often appears exaggerated to me. These patients, deprived of the physical capacities they once had or the ability to hold down a job, cathect their pain and lamentation to varying degrees (different levels of algosis). Are all somatic disorders psychosomatic, as some current theories appear to maintain?

The question must therefore be put differently and must examine the basic nature of psychosomatisation process. This is what I hope to have begun to do by comparing and contrasting the very early defences of psychosomatic patients (with somatic lesions) and their extreme opposites (psychogenics with no organic lesions).

The latter cathect outwards very early and reconstruct the mother, satisfying their ascendancy instinct and need for control, at the cost of a possible breakdown into pain. If this happens, they then find another paradoxical defence in the pain which gives equal protection against the stimuli. Cathected in action and then possibly in pain, the body is protected and remains so. They do not somatise in the sense in which I understand it, but psychosomaticians will not agree. By this I mean that they can contract the diseases that are part of human life, although this is rare, but they do not present with the "psychosomatic" picture which really gives the impression of a failing of the mind. It is in these patients that the classic characteristics described by the analysts of the Paris School mentioned earlier can really be observed.

The "psychosomatic" patient has not cathected his body. He has leapt to its defence but his fortress has been stormed, razed to the ground and left with little protection for its defence.

To summarise, my long experience with chronic pain sufferers has convinced me:

- In post-traumatic patients whose lesions due to the trauma are slight or non-existent, the hyperactivity that preceded it and the seemingly incurable pain that followed it are an affirmation of life.
- In psychosomatic patients, something has been lacking. Protection has failed. The stimulus barrier, by which I mean what is established as such in the mother-child relationship, has been overstretched and become mortified in its fight against too many stimuli.

Hypochondriacs, post-traumatic pain patients without lesions or with slight lesions and patients called psychosomatic with minor or very serious organic illnesses are the three compulsory reference groups in the world of pain. These patients are the boundaries of an area in which all chronic pain sufferers can be found: the injured and patients with physical symptoms who find it hard to bear their suffering. The table *Psychogenics and psychosomatics* (see next page) shows the similarities and differences between the three reference categories when their specific characteristics are strongest. For example, psychosomatics are seen in their moments of "operant life", as described by the psychosomaticians of Marty's school, which I think represents particular moments rather than the chronic norm. The term "Not applicable" refers to the fact that the aspect concerned does not appear spontaneously in the conversation.

PAIN, A SHIELD AGAINST A PSYCHIC STIMULUS

> "I wake up without anxiety but with palpitations of the heart. My alarm clock says 2 a.m." (Freud, 1900)

This is the end of one of Freud's dreams in which his son appeared. He was called up during the war and was then sent to the front and Freud had not had news of him for some time. We know that at the time Freud was suffering precardiac pains which worried him considerably. The dream was troubling enough to wake him but Freud experienced heart pain rather than anxiety. We remember what he said about Emmy von N., explaining that physical pain can prevent mental pain. The palpitations did not prevent Freud initiating psychic elaboration on "the hidden tendency that the feared death of my son might satisfy". We can see how the body has initially bypassed the psyche, protecting it from anxiety and psychic pain, and then the psychic elaboration has taken over.

This Freudian example shows how pain can form a shield against a psychic stimulus associated with an incompatible representation containing something painful. Can this be categorised as a hysterical conversion mechanism? In one sense yes, but it does not fulfil this role in this case. It is more accurate to say that there is a defensive function in pain, one often sought. We have seen it in action continuously in various psychic structures such as hypochondria and post-traumatic neuroses.

Table 1: Psychogenics and psychosomatics

Themes	Hypochondriacs	Psychogenic lumbalgics	Psychosomatics
Lesion	No	No	Yes
Complaint of pain	Yes	Yes	No
Knowledge	Existence of a theory	No knowledge	No knowledge
Temporality	Timeless	In two phases: past/present	No temporality
Feeling	Certainty	Certainty	Not applicable
Cause mentioned	No cause	Two causes: archaic/recent	No cause
Location	Anatomical/physiological scene	Organ or region	Diseased organ
Recital	Rich and repetitive recital	Colourful, repetitive and associative	Poor recital
Affect	Triumph or anxiety	Painful affect	Little affect
Psyche	Lively, often poetic	Dramatic	No dramatisation Operant thinking possible
Cathexis of the world	Split: normal/somatic	Split in time: hyperactivity/pain	Factual
Auto-eroticism	As a shield	In two acts	Not applicable
Mother	Preserved/controlled Faecalised	Idealised/to be repaired	Not applicable
Sense of guilt	No conscious sense of guilt	No conscious sense of guilt	Not applicable
Loyalty to the doctor	Potentially loyal	More or less loyal	Very loyal
Curability	Not curable by medication	Not curable by medication	Lesion curable by medication

But it can also play a part in some temporary states which place heavy stress on the restraining and elaborative capacity of the psyche. This is quite often the case with mourning. Some mourning is difficult or even impossible. There are many varieties of pathological mourning (mourning denied, mourning put aside, mourning overcathected and religiously preserved etc.). One of the forms that mourning can take is physical pain.

I have often seen patients come to the clinic after a referral by doctors who do not know what else to do. These people are very anxious and bring us a pain syndrome and piles of medical records: examinations, scans, MRI etc. – all negative. We soon learn the facts about a recent bereavement which the patient mentions but does not talk about. There is a touching identification with the person lost, but the split is such that the mention of an association between the loss and the illness makes no sense to the patient, who has regrouped and taken up a vigorously defended narcissistic position: he is ill. In cases like this the body nullifies the psychic suffering by its pain or limits it while representing it.

We have to be able to understand the mute appeal contained in the repeated expressions of pain by these subjects. It is an appeal for consolation. It presupposes a hard to perceive regression behind the activity deployed by patients who are assailed by diverse erratic physical sensations and are on the lookout for pathologies that their doctors keep dismissing. Their pain is topical and in actual fact external and it prevents an internal topic seen as dangerous or difficult from being expressed. The body helps the psyche. One patient who had been followed up for a while and was aware of the role of the diverse erratic pains in his avoidance of mourning said to me one day: "In the end I preferred suffering stupidly to intelligently!"

In all cases of cathexis of the body's pain, sensation is preferred to affect. A. Green said of the affect that it was a look at the emotional body. Looking assumes a degree of distancing from what is looked at. Sensation "does not look at itself"; it is content to be a feeling. This is the reason for preferring to choose pain, because the affect – look – would bring back undesirable representations and stimulate the psyche. When the cathexis of physical pain is firmly anchored in the psyche, what I call algosis, the position achieved is extremely robust. When the new system has become established, the stimulus is pain and the discharge of the stimulus is also pain. This circular game is very economical and automatically keeps the affect at a distance. Therefore this system is sound and reassuring and also achieves what is so important for a human being: expressing complaints with their dual function of appeal for help and assertion of the need for care. This type of organisation leaves the body unharmed, which we know is not the case with psychosomatic patients, whose bodies are affected but who express no complaints.

An article by M.-L. Roux (1984) on relaxation psychotherapy discusses this defensive recourse to the body and its sensations, mainly of pain. The traditional analytical structure ignores the body and uses language and free association to manage the play of the affects. M.-L. Roux talks about some patients (personality neuroses, borderline personality disorders) who often express complaints on a physical level. They refer to migraines, tachycardia, various algia, insomnia, pain spasms etc. She indicates that these patients (who are well known to us) organise their lives around the symptom "which isolates the painful part and allows a psychic life and an apparently normal life". The patients are divided. They develop under relaxation of the motor and sensory resistance built up against the appearance of the affects and emergence of the drive.

When they are asked to let go, i.e. to abandon their habitual motor defences, which goes against this "perceptive denial of their own physical states", they may exhibit resistance to perceiving what I would call "the healthy body". This resistance is reflected *inter alia* in "paradoxical sensations": pain, burning or minor sensory messages, but these are felt to be truly unbearable intrusions. What may also happen is the disappearance of sensory experience, rejection of feeling or escape from what is happening in the body, which is then replaced by social chitchat. The silent body certainly has plenty to say.

Little attention is paid to the fact that in modern life everyone uses pain as a pretext when they are criticised, even for something insignificant. This is what we hear: "I have a headache" or "I could not sleep last night" used as the first defence against attack. Children who have not done their homework say they feel sick, don't they? Small, brief algoses that occur between feeling and imagination, but they are genuine when they are expressed.

The following clinical case shows how the elaborative work that reawakened earlier mourning made a subject understand the defensive role of an organic pain that had no link with the mourning.

Madame L. An obdurate memory

I had been told that Madame L. was coming. I had been given a description of her many physical problems which was not encouraging. When she arrived, rather obese, on two crutches, with her oxygen bottle and tubes in her nostrils and her hesitant and clearly painful gait, I said to myself that the description had been accurate. Madame L. was a very nice woman, intelligent and extremely precise in her description of her woes: "generalised arthritis, the pain of which is aggravated by being overweight, as are the breathing difficulties".

She soon started talking about her past, her family and her childhood. The general idea was that she had never been able to do what she wanted: "I have always been thwarted". Her complaints, both physical and mental, were not excessive and were expressed with great concern for accuracy. She was one of the few people who asked me what my plan was to cure her, how it would be organised and what my prognosis was. I told her that she would only be able to understand my answer after several months working together and then there would be no need to ask. This humorous exchange pleased her and our understanding began.

In this situation I immediately adopted a strong parental position different from the one taken by the doctors who were powerless to cure her, and different also from the one taken by her parents in refusing to allow their daughter to take up her chosen profession. I literally prescribed for her the need for intensive and repeated respiratory rehabilitation. I projected an authoritarian and yet protective paternal image, thereby also projecting a particular quality on the transferential situation. Two factors emerged from this strong position: the inability of the doctors to keep her, although the rehabilitation proved very beneficial, and then above all the meaning of her failure to attend the rehabilitation which the doctors had recommended and she had not completed. Was it the expression of a totally unconscious and possibly fatal masochism? I had to question my intervention which was finally quite violent and which she felt to be intransigent. This case is a perfect example because it shows how far the transferential situation can be infiltrated by reality in the treatment of this type of patient. I was not neutral; I was a benevolent dictator. Obviously this behaviour leaves profound traces in the subsequent transference.

And the consequences were very favourable. It is not my custom to intervene on somatic matters, but it really appeared essential that I should. By the end of a few sessions I saw her arrive without oxygen, much less breathless and moving more freely. I had the impression that because she could breathe more easily and without assistance, a reaction that one might call euphoric had been triggered, enabling her to decathect the weight of her arthritic pain. Anyway, she improved and we continued from there, both being witnesses to her regrowth and improved pain situation – true psychotherapy. There is no need to discuss it here. I just want to say that it was achieved for my patient in a spirit of enthusiastic commitment. Once again, pain and its treatment had provided the opportunity for psychotherapy and I wonder why it had not been tried before.

I was pleased with the progress of the treatment and asked her one day if she would let me use her case for my research work. She interrupted and told me the following story:

- "A cousin of mine was the instructor of a group. My son was a member and was found dead by a waterfall. No-one knows what happened. My cousin was very traumatised and decided to write about it. He gathered stories and news together and wrote a pseudo imaginary account inspired by the incident to "exorcise" the emotion of the nightmarish experience. He felt better afterwards, unlike me. [...] In my case, I could not separate myself from the physical pain, unaware that it covered the old

> pain that had never scarred over. Coming here has made me rediscover it and even if I cannot get away from it, at least I can finally learn to live with it."

Pain, then, is just an evil to be fought. We must not confuse its disorganising effect with the defensive aspects which it can also take on. Recourse to physical pain is an archaic defence. It is the defence of the baby calling for its mother. It is the defence used to fight the annihilation anxieties experienced during early distressed states. These anxieties are called catastrophic and unnamed anxiety by some authors. Pain is better than annihilation. The sensation of pain is something known, certain and reliable and above all is a primal sensation, doubtless the first to give the feeling of existing. In the absence of anti-cathexis offered by the mother to allow the original repression, it is a position of withdrawal, a solution both simple and economic.

The fact that in some cases it resists all treatments and yields only after psychotherapy shows the wide range of its roles and functions. It is difficult to define them accurately because their paths cross. Pain is a many-sided and adaptable world which is always immediately burdened with the weight of masochism.

The painful libido is strongly adherent. When it takes possession of an organ or bodily function, which can happen to anyone (we all have our preferred territories, which can also be called our favourite weak points), it clings on and becomes a secure staging post. Like Freud's palpitations, they represent an easy discharge area, for example to accompany an initial anxiety and relieve it. This crude defence is the one operating - by different processes - in hypochondriacs, traumatic neurosis patients and many others.

It is organised and structured in or around something repetitive and known which is always reassuring. "The fact of rediscovering the known is marked by pleasure," says Freud, and it is "a saving on what is expended psychically". Both these aspects are important in some psychic organisations, especially when it is important to avoid the challenge of psychotherapy.

The revival by masochism of a pain cathected for some reason, or simply because it exists gives it considerable weight and resistance. The pain, an attempted solution like all the symptoms, is positioned between true healing and relapse. Nothing good and nothing bad can happen to me now. All this sums up the three main functions of pain, already mentioned but explained here more succinctly:

- The first lies in the establishment of strong narcissistic bases, assisted by colluding masochism. The subject auto-erotically savours his painful condition, sometimes ostentatiously and even provocatively. This attitude also allows and promotes the continuous deeply satisfying expression of the complaints. I shall define this aspect when discussing the reorganisation of the ego caused by pain.
- Just like obsessional behavioural defences such as hyperactivity or other defence mechanisms, physical pain can form an effective shield against a mental pain, which is experienced more intensely, or to bypass a psychic conflict that one wants to avoid. A stimulus barrier. This is the case with hysterics and we have seen cases of mourning avoided in this way.
- Finally, I am convinced that the "choice" of hyperactivity to combat the inherent distress is a defence against psychosomatic somatisation, despite the risk of sinking into the pain associated with it, although this is not necessarily the case. In my view it is not the pain that is protective, it is the inventive early cathexis of the outside world. Hyperactivity or some other defensive system, established instead of what I have called the mortification of the stimulus barrier which, having been rendered less effective, forbids the use of lateral cathexes with a defensive potential. An escape to the outside world instead of the fatal hammering of the stimuli.

Chapter 9

TREATING CHRONIC PAIN SUFFERERS[1]

> *"One has the impression of a force defending itself against healing by all means possible and determined to cling to the illness and suffering"*
> *Freud, "Analysis terminable and interminable"*

I want to try to show the specific problems involved in treating physical pain, and indicate the possible ways of disengagement from the painful cathexes, despite the pessimism of Freud's quotation.

All the patients I discuss were treated at the pain clinic described in detail in the appendix with a typical clinical example. They were all seen at every session first by one analyst and then by another, always in the same order[1].

Contrary to what might be thought after my emphasis on describing the three categories of pain sufferer (hysteria, hypochondria, post-traumatic neurosis) in which the psychogenic aspect is predominant and sometimes even represents the only cause of the pain, the number of patients

1 See the consultation procedures in the appendix

consulting us who present with organic disorders or post-traumatic somatic lesions is considerable. The numbers have even tended to increase in recent years and currently represent more than 65% of our patients. This is explained by the ever-increasing demands on hospital doctors, whose patients generally suffer from physical lesions.

They can be people suffering painful after-effects from surgery: to the thorax (heart or lungs), the vertebral, cervical or lumbar spine, various algodystrophies, painful scarring, neuropathic algia after plexus amputation or dilaceration (e.g. brachial), phantom limb pain, vascular algia of the face, trigerminal or other neuralgia, vascular pain in diabetics, dissection of the aorta or major blood vessels, pain following a trauma causing serious anatomical damage, after radiotherapy etc.

We have few patients with the alexithymic profile described by psychosomaticians because, as I said earlier, somaticians have no great problem dealing with them. Nevertheless we have seen a number of them and although it is true that some of them experience a period of depression and operant life and thinking, they do not all function in this way. With them the work is specific.

As regards our other – habitual - patients, we have to ask ourselves: Why do they turn to a pain clinic? And when they do, why do somaticians send them to us? Why has conventional medicine which is now so effective failed (this is the term used by the doctors)? And why are these patients often told by various doctors: "I can do nothing for you"? This is a serious problem in today's world. It will not be resolved by increasing the number of pain centres and clinics.

Doctors take the view that there is a disproportion in these patients between the pain they feel and the lesions they have, and that the same therapies used on equivalent patients work effectively.

The patients feel abandoned, do the rounds of the hospitals, have innumerable tests done, seek out alternative therapies and finally end up with us at the end of their tether. We sometimes feel like the dustbin of medicine and even of other more conventional pain clinics, because the virtues of sleight-of-hand smacking slightly of heresy are attributed to ours, run only by psychoanalysts. But patients and doctors are in agreement on two points.

They suffer too much. But then opinions diverge: for failings of diagnosis or therapy, say the patients; for purely imaginary reasons which have nothing to do with anatomical/ physiological disorders, think the doctors.

None of the many therapies tried (based on international consensus, add the doctors) has had any effect.

One can understand that if pain is an attempt at healing, or is at least capable of being firmly integrated in the psyche because the subject finds a meaning unknown to him, it is hard to imagine how it can be dislodged from a system chosen as the best available. Our experience has shown, however, that many of our patients have been able to develop, to abandon the position of refuge that their suffering represents and to reposition themselves on new foundations. They have succeeded in either managing their pain better by cathecting it less, or in the best cases being free of it altogether.

SOMATIC OR PSYCHOGENIC AETIOLOGIES

The aetiology of pain, somatic or psychogenic, is irrelevant. I wrote in detail earlier about the clinical study of hysteria, post-traumatic neuroses and hypochondria because these three categories are pure forms of the psyche's capacity to create pain and above all because they are prototypes. The work they require when the psychotherapist takes charge of them is the model to be followed in the treatment of patients whose suffering has an organic cause. A complex which is the cause of psychogenic pain and has the same function as a lesion responsible for pain due to an organic cause has the same characteristics. The former is essential to the economy of the psyche generating it because of its basic function of defence. The latter is itself chronically established (scarring, or progressive form) because it has triggered a chronic pain.

And the narcissistic wound accompanying the physical disease is certainly felt in the psyche. The mind sinks into pain with the body. When pain takes hold, its modus operandi is the same.

Everything depends on the quality of the subject's previous cathexes. I recall a patient operated on for a lumbar discopathy responsible for paralysing hyperalgic sciatica who had another hyperalgic crisis in the regression phase of the intervention. He told me how one night, which he called that "terrible night", he passed the time trying to make a plan for a meeting he had to go to. But the pain seemed to return even more strongly and ruined his attempts. He would start again and would again be gripped by the pain. All night he tried to overcome the misery he felt and wondered what he would have done if he had not had an urgent meeting to prepare for. An example of acute pain such as this gives us a kind of sped-up version of what happens when chronic pain takes root, and shows the essential part that distraction can play.

A real conflict is set up between the pre-existing psychic cathexes and those imposed by the reality of the pain. It all depends on what has been built up throughout the subject's past and the topography of his current cathexes. Adherence to the important basic cathexes, giving the structure of the ego its robustness, will form an effective defence against invasion by pain and leave greater space for that invasion, unlike labile narcissistic or object cathexis. I must emphasise that I am not talking here of pusillanimous or soft subjects. They are not "pain sufferers," they have a particular attitude towards pain – an exaggerated imaginary fear. They often prove to be surprisingly stoical when they suffer a hyperalgic affliction.

Patients who attend a pain clinic represent a very small proportion of chronic pain sufferers. Most of them confide their sufferings to their doctors, and with them somehow take the difficult path that pain involves, without feeling the need to consult algologist "specialists". In the rheumatology department where I worked, I once had occasion to see a

Beaujolais wine grower suffering from chronic lumbar sciatica with acute episodes whose X-rays showed the terrible physical damage caused by arthritis and his work. Despite this, the man continued looking after his vines, kneeling on a doormat, and hardly ever stopped working: "Have to prune vines properly!" he said in his Burgundian dialect, but he would never dream of using the excuse of his continual pain to leave the medical environment of the hospital – which he might have thought unsatisfactory – and consult other doctors specialising in pain.

Similarly, patients with rheumatoid arthritis, an extremely painful and typically psychosomatic condition, were never a problem for the doctors in the department. Although they were all aware of my presence as a pain specialist, they never asked to meet me. I must say that I was very surprised by this and wondered, at least initially, why the lumbalgics who had next to nothing wrong with them suffered so much and yet the patients with deformed joints and movements restricted by the disease and the pain did not complain, or rather complained in ways that were logical and were accepted by the doctors. The therapeutic alliance was not broken. I had the opportunity to meet enough patients with rheumatoid arthritis to realise that after a certain time the mourning for the previous good health was completed and the disease and the pain that went with it were integrated even if not accepted.

Freud wrote (in *Beyond the Pleasure Principle*) that when there was a post-traumatic organic lesion, the traumatic neurosis did not take hold. We cannot say that this is confirmed nowadays, but he showed an intuition that separated the somatic reality from the reality of the pain. The absence of lesion may trigger the painful neurosis, but patients suffering lesions such as arthritis prove that the reverse can be true and the lesion does not necessarily cause the neurosis. But to the somatician, the pain has to prove its organic origin. This is why the cases of the wine grower and arthritic patients satisfy medical logic. But all the patients called psychogenic, whom I discussed at length in the first part, indicate the need for a nosography that differs from the conventional one for an understanding of patients in chronic pain.

I have just contrasted psychosomatic patients who have painful lesions but complain little, with psychogenic pain sufferers whose lesions are few or non-existent but who complain a great deal. Between these two extremes are all the possible processes of response to pain, whether lesional or not.

PSYCHOANALYSIS AND PSYCHOTHERAPY

Pain is not a drive; it has neither a direct goal nor an object. It cannot be repressed. Freud called it a *pseudo* drive and to combat it saw only the process of distraction which, seen as such, could only be a temporary solution. But like a drive it imposes a need for work on the psyche and profoundly reorganises it. This means that the spontaneous evolution of the subject's psyche is modified, and deformed by the mourning it involves, and the chronic trauma it represents. The psychoanalyst must therefore be able to offer patients in pain an area of work to which he is accustomed.

This cannot be psychoanalysis. But we shall see that thanks to language the patient himself finds "the path of the lost memories", as Freud said. We shall also see how this language develops and becomes fertile and enriched. But the patient does not come to see us wanting analysis. He expresses a need: the need to be relieved of his pain. But our attitude is analytical. The kind of conversation that we have from the first encounter, consisting of listening and paying attention but without the questioning that patients expect makes them realise that something different from usual is happening. They are particularly struck by the fact that we do not examine them.

We conceal nothing from them but do not explain our methods. They join spontaneously in the diet of words that we offer them. The amazing thing is that their discourse adapts quite quickly even if it is mainly descriptive and factual at the beginning. Unlike what Freud says about his hysterical patients, when the conversation involves the pain symptoms these patients forget their pain and accept a narrativity very like "free association"(a basic rule of analysis), with at least the structure of analysis but also with our help and complicity.

Our desire is not to cure but to keep the patient, offer him a system that he will adopt and make him "like" our treatment so that he will come back and be interested in the sessions. Our work is rarely or never interpretative, but we often construct, offer information and links and facilitate inter-systemic psychic exchanges. Therefore no *furor sanandi*. We are aiming for integration of the pain into the patient's psyche. The idea being that the energy it has attracted to it has to be redistributed and replaced within the trauma sequence of the subject and his history.

The considerable but limited development (as Balint said) achieved by our patients is indicated by the often surprising and unexpected changes in their narrative. Our occasionally active support must have some therapeutic value for the pain. Does it offer a cure? The impression we have been given by the majority of patients of slowly escaping from the straitjacket of pain, undergoing a kind of metamorphosis and cathecting life differently is enough for us. A cure for human pain is surely a myth?

Madame R. A polyphony of pain

I describe this complex case by way of an example, but one which is representative and shows how physical pain and personality disorders can defend each other in turn, in a dizzy to-ing and fro-ing, whereas the serious psychosomatic problem falls silent and a cause cannot be determined. Also noticeable is the heterogeneity of discourse which contains dreams and childhood memories but also a "traumatic" part, full of nightmares and horrible daydreams, all co-existing in a striking context combining love and hate.

Madame R. was a 50 year old woman who came to see us eight months after a car accident in which she had been seriously injured: cranial trauma with a skull fracture, loss of consciousness, 23 centimetre scalp, 18 stitches and fractures to the right hand, arm, knee and foot. She complained of amnesia of old memories but thought about her accident constantly, which made her cry. She dreamed about it at night and in colour relived a wheel racing towards her. She would wake up in a state of acute anxiety. She also complained of headaches, dizziness and pain in her arm, knee and foot. When recounting the circumstances of the accident, she insistently repeated the vision of the motorcycle wheel that had shattered the front right-hand door and entered the car, pushing back the seat she was sitting on – a wheel that she said grew larger as it approached and would cut her into pieces, as she said. She was very angry with the motorcyclist and even more so because all the blame had been put on her husband who was driving and had had his driving licence taken away. She told me:

- "And he died as well, that..., after flying twelve metres! He shouldn't have been going fast! Where did he come from? He wasn't there because my husband had not seen him!"

After describing her accident to me several times, Madame R. curiously recounted a dream about a father-in-law (her mother's second husband) who would not reappear in her conversation until more than two years later. In this dream the father-in-law had urinated into a box in her presence. She added that it was a recurring dream. She then associated on her dramatic life story. Her father had been a stallholder liked by, and attractive to women, a "bon viveur" who liked a drink. He only returned to the house to beat her mother and preside over a reign of terror. They were poor and had nothing. She had been brought up by childminders until she was 4 and had not long returned to her mother before she was packed off to her maternal grandparents. Her mother was very cruel and broke her leg one day when putting on her shoe.

Madame R. then changed the subject to her other somatic misfortunes and I learned that she had had asthma, chronic bronchitis, pulmonary tuberculosis with many relapses and breast cancer for which she was due to have another operation. She then resumed talking about her mother for whom no words could be hard enough. I learned that she had also been in the car on the day of the accident and was given some idea of the exchanges between the two women. When Madame R. mentioned some time after the accident that she had been seriously injured, her mother replied "with a superior air":

- "And I am a widow!
- "So I am nothing!" concluded Madame R.

To each her narcissism.

I learned all that in our first conversation and was astonished by the words of this woman who introduced me to three aspects of her suffering at the same time. Firstly her post-traumatic neurosis with physical pain and visions of the accident day and night. Then her litany of numerous serious somatic disorders which some narcissistic need drove her to list. Finally, I saw her afflicted by what would prove to be a borderline personality disorder with its violence directly entirely against her mother. She engaged with her throughout her treatment in a relationship of true-false love and true-false hatred that joined the two of them as if with barbed wire. This was what I said to her one day and it was one of the rare interventions that had the merit of mobilising her somewhat. I wondered what the therapy profile could possibly be for such a combination of different psychic problems. I had the impression of a complex maze, but divined the defensive function it might have and the need for this.

Mme. L. had immediately incorporated her current trauma into her original trauma, fusing her physical and mental complaints, those associated with the accident and those she had always had. She used one as a defence against the other. Even during a conversation, if what she was relating about her past was too terrible, she would suddenly be seen to grimace, complain about her arm and start rubbing it. I sometimes said to myself that the accident had enabled her to undergo psychotherapy that she would never have asked for otherwise. But her mentally painful evocations of the past revived her physical pain of the present. She was difficult to follow up. The regression caused by the trauma and pain had reawakened the old demons.

Rather against my expectations, Mme. R. proved to be an extremely loyal patient who never missed a session. The need to talk was superimposed on the need to get better which had brought her to us. She was quite a nice person, but following her as she juggled with the three problems discussed above gave me headaches. As time passed things became clearer and a conventional borderline personality disorder programme was arranged, but was often affected by the sudden return of her physical suffering and traumatic neurosis: pains, recurrence of the traumatic nightmares and visions, preoccupation with her lungs or cancer, and during heated moments when she could no longer control the violence towards her mother. We saw how the body could come to the rescue of a submerged psyche in two ways, by means of the physical pain or the anxiety of the disease.

Madame R., whose mother had gone back to the East, brought her back to her own city and found her somewhere to live nearby. It was a duel to the death between the two women. I was only there to take my patient's ferocious complaints about her mother, as a kind of witness from whom she required, above all, agreement. I had no means of intervening. The antidepressive aspect of her violence was obvious. Because of this triumph over her mother, represented by the "legitimacy" of complaints confirmed by the somatic reality, the depression could not emerge. Madame R. was slowly discharging. However, her mother tired of this adversarial relationship and decided to go back East, but with a plan which literally destroyed her daughter: she intended to go back to her first husband whom she wanted as a "companion and lover" and refused to allow her daughter to resume any contact with her father. "She would even deny me that!" the daughter said to me.

At that precise moment she again sought refuge in the body and the pain and arranged many more consultations with doctors. But the return of the headaches, pains and insomnia was not enough and Madame R. became quite depressive. Although she had been doing quite well until

> then, sustained by her aggressive attitude towards her mother, she sank into an almost melancholic apathy on the very day of her departure. That adversary who was just as resolute as her daughter had succeeded in touching the precise sensitive and above all painful spot.
>
> The situation became oedipian even if the problem was not. The appeal to the mother at the time of the pain had been unheard and the approach to the father meant: "Look how my mother treats me!"
>
> Our consulting room was the theatre of war between the two women who fought over their love of the same man. Madame R. decided to go and see what was happening for herself. Her journey was even more eventful that I could have imagined and I heard all about it when she returned. In a way unhoped for, the conflict took a new turn due to its love triangle aspect and despite the rivalry, Madame R. met her father again. I was particularly impressed by one episode which was moving: her father had given his daughter a small box and told her that he had always kept it with the idea of giving it to her. Madame R. was touched, clasped it to her heart and wept. She said no more about her pain and began making plans with her husband. A spark had been lit. Our therapy had provided an area of discharge or holding structure with solid walls, an accompaniment to form links and offer cautious hypotheses, above all a survival. Madame R. had been able to internalise more reliable and peaceable parental imagos and had become more skilled at self-consolation.

This example highlights the adaptable flexibility and functionality of physical pain and also its limits. Suffering to avoid thinking, suffering to avoid being depressed (up to a point, as we have seen) or to repress over-explosive violence, and suffering also to legitimise a necessity, a need for complaint, which is essential for narcissistic affirmation. Was the total disappearance of the patient's "psychosomatic" syndromes (asthma, bronchitis, tuberculosis, cancer) related to our long period of psychotherapy? I cannot say. The somaticians were proposing to operate on the cancer again when our patient had her accident. No more was said about it. We should also note that the patient immediately fused her three painful problems into a single complaint which was essential for her.

Therefore, although the psychotherapy undertaken by patients in pain can be monotonous at the beginning, it can extricate itself from this monomania to tackle extraneous problems. We see old problems emerge and old wounds reappear. Sibling rivalries, childhood sexual abuse reviving a strong sense of guilt, or memories of wrongs committed in the past and giving a meaning to the pain through remorse. Mental pain forgotten or repressed emerges as a result of the physical pain but restores unity to the patient, who can then more easily position the trauma of the pain within the sequence of previous traumas.

Whatever the origin or aetiology of their suffering, the patients who consult us express their pain in the present tense and also in the perfect tense, which is the present past: "I have been operated on ... I have had an accident ... or I feel discharges ... I suffer from morning till night." These two conjugations are those of catastrophe.

Then they move to the imperfect, a sensitive form, not to capture the past but to revive it gently and move the doctor. The imperfect guards against the decisive future, it is the time before the pain, a time that no longer exists. It is a nostalgic time which, as we shall see, is also the time of hope because it expresses the paradise lost. The time afterwards is the time of pain. By articulating these two times individually, the grammar can separate them from the present neurosis which is the pain.

The experience of patients locked in pain is a depressive one. The depression is caused by the acute feeling of loss of what they could do before and will never be able to do again, and above all loss of the ability to cathect anything other than the pain.

The failure to be cured is like an abandonment. A mother appealed to who does not come. This is the "appeal" dimension of their suffering. The over-cathexis of an organ, a function or a part of the body can become painful if it combines with an experience of the mother's absence, when the representation of that absence has been unable to develop adequately. Ferenczi referred to a confusion of language between parents and children when the language of tenderness meets the language of passion. I have often had this impression when listening to patients and their despair at never having been heard. Doctors and patients sometimes speak foreign languages.

PAINFUL NEONARCISSISM

When the body/psyche is invaded by the heavy artillery of physical pain, it regresses. Physical pain brings profound and lasting changes to the psyche and a need to work through it of a particular kind, regressive and restrictive. It is important to understand these changes in order to achieve the essential empathy with the patients, and help them escape gradually and by means of their own processes from the vicious circle of despair. It is important to emphasise again that the origin of the pain does not affect its treatment. However, the counter-transferential position of the psychoanalyst is modified by the level of intensity of the pain or the gravity of the somatic situation (patients at the end of their lives, incurable pathologies).

We need to be able to listen to the characteristics of this painful neonarcissism, how the patient bears it and what he says about it. He has been unable to make this heard previously or elsewhere. The depressive part of his ego is affected. The source of the drive represented by the lost object has disappeared and has been replaced by pain. If the drive object was a projection of the self into the world due to a deficiency of narcissistic libido connection, its disappearance is a disaster. It causes emptiness. The object and the self have broken down together. A Basque pelota player without a wall to hit his ball to cannot carry on playing. This gives the idea of a strategy for this kind of problem: to re-establish or reinvent a playing field.

The subject is faced with an image different from himself and wounded by pain. The strata on which the narcissism was based have wavered and are outdated and useless. Everything depends, of course, on the previous psychic organisation. I have met a similar situation with top sportsmen at the end of their careers. Some accept an end which was inevitable. They have prepared for it and are organised, planning to become coaches for example. Others cling on too long, want to show that they are still around and experience what they feel to be downfall or rejection.

Pain certainly kills everything. The few flights of the psyche towards a world beyond pain are paradoxically painful in themselves because they soon come back to earth and force the subject back into his impotence. They are only illusions and just leave the chronic pain sufferer with a bitter taste in the mouth. Therefore this painful neonarcissism tends to be self-maintained and self-aggravated, which justifies Freud's position in *Beyond the Pleasure Principle*. If the pain becomes the narcissistic overtension referred to by J. Cournut, the entire Ego becomes painful, leading to the continuous over-cathexis of the pain which naturally brings the masochistic attitude of the patient into play. We know that masochism and narcissism are closely related. In the 1914 article Princeps which introduces narcissism, Freud uses the examples of pain, disease, hypochondria, sleep, paraphrenia etc.

The new narcissism that has taken hold is not just content to enjoy the suffering in silence, in an autoeroticism satisfied only by masochism. Aggression and sadism, masochism's old partners, are there, ready to manifest themselves. This can be through the implacable expedient of depression, as the patient's family will strongly maintain, or it can be through presence responses, vigorous protests denying impotence, or it can be through the monotonous and repetitive litany of complaints, especially if the complaints of today reopen the old wounds of the subject's past and particularly his childhood. But it can also be an expression of the violence of injured narcissism reproaching the mother-doctor for not looking after and healing him. It sometimes happens, though rarely, that in mid conversation the patient is gripped by a fit of rage fuelled by his feelings of impotence and loss and attacks his interlocutor, physically if he feels the need.

Another apparently paradoxical expression of painful neonarcissism consists of an affirmation of the painful disorder and its incurability. The patient finds new prestige in the failure of all the doctors he has seen. I repeat that we come at the end of the road (the last chance) after a long medical journey full of disappointments:

- "I have seen such and such a doctor, I have been to such and such an institution, I have tried all the possible treatments: it has done me no good!"

The patient is narcissised masochistically because he is the one who suffers most in the world, no-one listens to him, his pain resists everything that the medical world can offer him. And behind these sometimes emotionally disturbed assertions we can clearly hear unspoken but explicit words such as: "You can do what you want, you will never cure me". At times like these we must not forget that the model that must appear like a watermark or backdrop in the recesses of our mind is the mother model. These violent calls to order, which are demands for reparation from the impossible ideal mother, must be heard and registered in the therapist's psyche to give them an acknowledgement and so that the engrams they leave provide a return for the therapy later. The sufferer has been recognised. Perhaps we should now bring in a concept developed by D. Rosé (1997), that of primal endurance, the experience of the therapist in these circumstances. It ought to enable him somehow to tolerate a violence which will leave its potentially usable mark but not lead to retaliation. We can also recall the primal violence of P. Aulagnier and the distancing that allows the child and the mother to adapt, which she calls a conjunction. One has to surprise the patient, not only by this kind of reaction to his violence but also by an attitude of togetherness to make a difference to his psyche.

I must emphasise what I call the need for complaint and making oneself heard, an expression of the painful narcissism with its strong sadistic component. As I said about lumbalgics, patients want to make us experience what they have lived through and relive what they have suffered, and they demand that we be the ideal fix-it: mothers that they have often not known. They want to be great examples of suffering and failure. As Freud said: the patient "is so to speak fixed in the trauma ... unless evoking the enigmatic masochistic tendencies of the ego" (1920). The pain drives the complaint. The need for complaint drives the pain. This need for complaint is what distinguishes algetic patients, the pain neurotics who come to see us in large numbers, from the others: the uncomplaining pain sufferers who often carry lesions and whose scope for improvement is often - but not always - much less.

There is a split, particularly in the former, between the part that wants to heal and the narcissistic part enhanced in status by the pain. The therapist has to be able to survive. It is important for him to discover the strata on which the old narcissism was built, now split in Manichean fashion from the painful narcissism. Both are over-cathected, the first in nostalgia and the second through masochism. The body "cured" of the pain will be a "reassembled" body.

WHEN REGRESSION REMEMBERS

The period of pain is also the period of regression. In "Body Image", Shilder maintains that this regression is dual, anal and narcissistic, and entails recourse, which is also a return to magical thoughts. Freud said, quoting V. Bush (1914): "The world shrinks to the narrow gap of the molar". A "painful myopia" exists. The objects are close, the remote is inaccessible. This spatial regression is only one aspect of a profound and temporal regressive process. It is easy to talk of regression but more difficult to define it in metapsychological terms. I would say that chronic pain sufferers rediscover a world of affects, fears and limitations once experienced or similar to what they once knew. They have strong feeling of dependence, impotence and despair that this should be so. It is a world evoking that of childhood, which is why I refer to regression, but which is also suffused by the experience of loss and above all tormented by pain.

A child does not live in the past; it lives in hope. Its megalomania imagines a destiny which is illusory and variable but always plausible and it marvels at its illusions. The pain sufferer is not a child. He knows that he is an adult and does not see himself in the future. The doctor has the authority of a parent and the patient is passive. Going back into the hands and under the authority of the "grown-ups" is often felt as a wound to the narcissism, paradoxically compounded by the fact that the "grown-ups" are useless. All patients experience this regression but accept it willingly when the objective – healing – appears easily achievable or at least possible. This is not the case with our patients. We are their last chance, but in chronic pain, as the word implies, there is nothing to say that the period of suffering will end.

Some patients do manage to cathect it minimally and their Ego is scarcely "impoverished", to use Freud's expression. Their self-esteem is saved, they accept their limitations and are capable of continuing to cathect beyond the pain. Above all they are capable of mourning. I remember a lady who "profited", as she said, from her pain and inactivity to write her memoirs as a member of the Resistance and pass them on to a young relative. With her the work was easy.

But generally the patient's regressive psyche does not have the resources to overcome the regression through thought and certainly not to experience it for itself in order to make something of it, for example by anti-cathecting it.

Regression can also mean that when the psyche is overwhelmed by almost obsessional thoughts (pain never lets itself be forgotten), it frustrates or even paralyses the associative abilities, and the inventive work of elaboration which allows the system to breathe due to the simple connections between the agencies. Mental function is no longer the same. Fantasies are nothing more than empty desires. In short, the psyche undergoes a hard resistance battle that absorbs and impoverishes it.

Regression is therefore the ally and perhaps the motor of the reversal of the drive energy to the ego brought about by means of the pain. As far as our patients are concerned, for a long time I saw this and the other changes in their ego only as a consequence of their painful state, but this did not seem adequate to fully encompass the clinical condition. The concept of regression is not a simple one. I cannot imagine that it consists of a return journey leading from one psychic position to another earlier one, following the same path.

Clinically we can see things like this: a regressive process occurs initially, for example due to the pain. Owing to this process, old fixations are revived and rekindled, but the important thing is that the regression finds its place, i.e. it goes to a previous non-random position. It is not just a defensive withdrawal; it has an ambivalent *intent* serving both the life and the death instincts.

A. Fine advances a similar idea in his fine article "Regression as organiser". He quotes Freud (*Beyond the Pleasure Principle*):

> "The sole nature of instinct lies in regression and the sole difference between, for example, the life and death instincts lies in the end of the regression." (Fine, 1992)

I think that like the traumatic dream this is a return to a past situation of failure or non-accomplishment, a situation of refusal or impotence, which has given rise to a fixation by default, so to speak. The regression is the opportunity for a second chance offered to an unsatisfied desire which has a strongly ambivalent aim combining conflicting valences linked by masochism. It is a blend of masochistic satisfactions and those giving what is normally called pleasure. This is a form of trauma fixation, an area of enjoyment. Pain quite naturally takes the place of a goal for a desiring force which has vague forms.

Fine refers to "an ontogenetic process with growth from an economic point of view which indicates regression as a consequence not a cause of the unravelling and as a drive towards Eros not Thanatos." (*ibid.*)

I lean towards Eros and Thanatos merged, which seems compatible to me with what we imagine pain can bring to a regressive psyche. Pain, a borderline personality disorder between passivity and activity, certainly merges victim and torturer, but it is a guarantor and witness of life. Representing a regressive solution for the psychogenic pain sufferer, it can compel recourse to that solution when it is caused by the injury or disease, especially if the patient has experienced distress, suffering and lack of consolation in his history or prehistory which have left engrams. The masochistic turmoil inherent in the reality of the past, generated from an initial pain stimulus, whether it is back pain, somatic compliance or a painful organic process, causes the psyche to use whatever fuel is available to achieve an old desire. Physical pain can be a reminder of the prehistoric or historic event and an attempt at another anachronistic appeal for help. This is the cause of the algetic hypercathexis. Regression is thus a return to the object. There is an instinctive attraction towards a forgotten traumatic position which somehow represents the object. If the regression has a goal and is a process that can be creative and energetic, it opens up means of psychotherapy for the patient. It is both a recall and a repetition, the only possible starting points from which to reverse the centripetal magnetic force of the pain and offer sources of rerouting or diversion, the only means of escaping the process of pain according to Freud.

REPETITION

There are many ways of repeating. Pain itself, in the unending process in which it is both stimulus and discharge of the stimulus, is a slow repetition beyond the bounds of time. The trauma causes the repetition. Some "traumatophilic" subjects seem to be demoniacally pursued by fate and repeat or see themselves repeating circumstances, events or accidents. This was the case with my patient Victor who repeated accidents or scenes marked by the same persistent scenario and then, after the pain had taken hold and he had lost control and activity, narration of the scenes of his accidents.

Monsieur T. Persistent fate

Monsieur T. had already had six car accidents resulting in cranial trauma, loss of consciousness or comas of varying lengths when I saw him for the first time. The periods of unconsciousness differed in duration, but sometimes became comas, the longest of which lasted for three weeks. I saw him after his seventh accident when he came out of a three-day coma. It would not be his last, I know of eleven in all, always in his boss's car, never his own. A sort of protocol had been established. Whenever he had an accident the emergency services would transfer him to the neurological hospital as soon as possible and give me a call to let me know: "Monsieur T. is back, you can go and see him". His last accident, the eleventh, was different, not being an accident at work. His boss had lent the patient one of his cars, an old American model, because his own had broken down, so that he could go to Italy on holiday. And 100 km from Lyon, bang! Accident, cranial trauma and coma ...

He was my patient for five of his eleven accidents and the process was always the same. He told the story of his accident but without many details or too much repetition. He spoke lightly and sometimes humorously of it. He said the worst thing was the nightmares or daytime thoughts and visions when he relived the accident. He said much more about headaches and dizzy spells but they never lasted for long. He related details of his daily life and provided some information on his earlier life as a child in Italy. He described a terrible father, feared by the many children in the family and related the sad life of a very poor family. "Padre padrone", he told me.

He thought I was kind, as was his boss: The proof: He had lent him his old American car, now a wreck, a car that could have been a collector's item, he added, with no apparent sense of guilt. His recital was fluent. He liked coming to see me, it did him good. Then, better, he would

> go back to work and a few months later crash another car or van belonging to the boss he liked.
>
> Nothing in our conversations could ever upset his unshakeable psyche: he had had an accident. He was suffering. He was getting better. He was going back to the job he loved (delivery man). He felt no aggression, was neither guilty nor responsible. "It is fate" he smiled. Monsieur T. understood nothing and especially not that the last accident had prevented a meeting with his father. Padre padrone only existed for me.

I have often had occasion to quote this case. It always provokes a sort of comedy of repetition. But it raises questions for me: All the accidents were serious (repeated loss of consciousness and coma). None threatened the patient's life or health. The implacable "fate" of their recurrence was therefore precautionary. I ask myself how once the patient had become embroiled in the behavioural neurosis, he managed to save his life every time and could so often reach the extreme point where the demoniacal force of the repetition was combined with the self-preservation instinct in his weird drawn games, without after-effects, residual pain or lessons learned from experience. The eleventh accident was the last, but I do not know what effect our work together had on the disappearance of the traumatic need. It is certainly the purest case of repetitive compulsion that I have ever seen.

Traumatic memories that return suddenly and violently revive the psychic cathexis of the sensation of pain, just as the sensation promotes the emergence of painful memories and images. The even more violent nightmares and the almost visual traumatic visions of the scene or an "excessively clear" (*überdeutlich*) part of the scene are another means of repetition. These phenomena may occur in conjunction with another kind of recollection, the common memory.

> I saw a lady whose husband had died in a condition of cachexia after a long and painful illness. She sometimes "saw" him, always in the same sequence that occurred "without warning", staggering along trying to walk and

> groaning with pain. The violence of these clear visions of the dying man trying to stay alive caused her great anxiety tinged with a powerful sense of guilt. It made her stomach churn. She reproached herself with not having helped him enough, particularly as she had hidden the truth from him when she was told belatedly how serious his illness was.
>
> But she could also let her thoughts stray to memories of her life with her husband, tenderly. She could then be reminded of the same traumatic scenes without feeling unbearable anxiety. The psychic elaboration took away the violence of the trauma. Trauma prevents elaboration, and that is one of its definitions. It is not so rare to see these two contradictory worlds coexisting. We can immediately see that in one case one is active and thinks and in the other one is passive and suffers: the mind is struck down. This is the difference between traumatic memory and screen memory.
>
> The psychic function differs according to whether it receives a screen memory or suffers a traumatic reminder, whatever its form. The woman I have just mentioned experienced an authentic traumatic neurosis which haunted her during the day in terrible quasi-hallucinatory perceptions and during the night in nightmares. No elaboration was possible. But the outpouring of her thoughts led back to gentler images which she readily evoked despite her distress. They helped her rediscover the affective world that she had lost through associations that diluted her pain. She completed her mourning.

There is a contradiction here which is not absolute because we have just seen these two opposite worlds coexisting. Patients in pain are traumatised by the pain itself, associated with a circumstance or event that is also traumatic. The outpourings of their thoughts are locked into the repetitive traumatic regression which is not conducive to elaboration. This state can be called traumatic but is also characterised either by the poverty of the memories, particularly the screen memories, or by the fact that they are not, or hardly ever, operant.

MEMORIES, SCREEN MEMORIES, TRAUMATIC MEMORIES

> "Behind the first memory of the emergence of the fetish is a submerged, forgotten phase of sexual development which is represented (*vertreten*) by the fetish as if by a "screen memory", the residue and fallout of which consequently form "the fetish"." (Freud, 1905)

Many small cumulative traumas allow the human psyche to be formed. What would become of us if the drive found its object? What would we be without the frustration, the *Versagung*, the "refusal" of J. Laplanche? Do we not confuse all these small psychic traumas that shaped our compliance with life with what may really have been traumatic for us? We should not forget that it was with reference to traumatic neurosis that Freud postulated hysteria and therefore simply neurosis at the beginning of his article and that he changed his theory to the point of overturning it by introducing repetition and the death instinct. I repeat that it can be no coincidence that he uses physical pain as an example of trauma.

The screen memory that comes back to the mind and the traumatic scene that forcibly breaks into it have some common features. Both are the fallout of past history and both are marked by their excessively clear representation. But it is their differences that are important and which define them.

The often anodyne aspect of the screen memory contrasts with its insistent reappearance in the psyche, a curious exception to childhood amnesia. It has a great capacity to be recalled and a totally neutral content. We know that it is a compromise formation, like the symptom, and that it is extremely condensed while being the result of displacements. As such, it is suitable for psychoanalysis and in transference is a generator of meaning. "Whenever in a memory the actual person of the *dreamer* enters the scene", Freud tells us (making a slip of the pen with the word dreamer when he is referring to a memory), "one can lay claim to this opposition between the acting ego and the remembering ego as if a childhood engram had been retranslated to a later time." (Freud, 1896).

In the same text he emphasises two fundamental points:

> "In a screen memory one sees oneself ... as if one were an observer outside the scene. One was at the centre of the situation and was not paying attention to oneself but to the outside world." (*ibid.* p. 113)

And elsewhere he expresses the idea "that we easily establish bridges which interconnect in all directions". In short, as the fruit of the psyche, the screen memory is suitable for psychotherapy.

The fact of seeing oneself in the scene, which involves duality in the subject or a kind of *split* (I use the word advisedly) between an observing part and an observed part, represents one of the functions of the ego: self-observation. Freud already highlighted this in "Outline of a Scientific Psychology", noting that the ego "sees" itself at work. But in the screen memory one sees oneself in the past with the eyes of the present, which introduces temporality and historicity and involves some kind of staging and work of the mind.

Trauma produces an altogether different split by striking down the unprepared, frightened ego. We saw in the chapter on hypochondria the Freudian and Ferenczian views of trauma. Event, reality and exterior all have various ways of being traumatic. Freud began with the sexual trauma of hysterics and moved on to war neuroses and then to "early wounds to the ego" in Moses in 1938. In relation to pain, which may originate from a trauma and is itself a trauma, we can observe its shattering effect on the ego. The ego becomes repetitive and the memory of the trauma does not have the features of the screen memory. In lumbalgics for example, we saw that the causal accident results in identical repetition of the narrative of the scene in which it occurred. And the patient does not see himself in his narrative. He is there. He cannot occupy an outside position. We play that role. We shall see later how the experience of psychotherapy can lead them to that previously impossible self-observation.

Lumbalgics are typical because their misery is or becomes an after-shock of the original distress which they narrate so easily. The slight trauma causing the pain is full of the trauma of that distress, just as the screen memory is filled with the earlier repressions of childhood. But there the resemblance stops. The catastrophic experiences of infancy and the childhood that followed have shaped a bruised, undeveloped or poorly developed ego.

Winnicott's posthumous article "Fear of breakdown" was published in the edition of the *New Journal of Psychoanalysis* (1974, No. 11) entitled "Impressions of emptiness". He talks about primitive agonies, anxiety not being a strong enough word to describe them. He lists some of them:

- Return to a non-integrated state
- Constant falling
- Loss of psychosomatic collusion
- Loss of a sense of reality and the ability to establish a rapport with the objects

He then adds that this is a way of repeating these primitive agonies. Winnicott's patients tended to be more psychotic than mine, particularly the lumbalgics. But I have used the term "melancholia of the body" about them, which must denote emptiness. Emptiness that repeats itself. Winnicott stresses this:

> "I maintain that clinical fear of breakdown is *fear of a breakdown that has already been experienced*[1]. Fear of the original agony." (*ibid.*)

"It is easier for a patient to recall a trauma than to remember that nothing happened when it could have happened," writes Winnicott. This sentence denotes the lack. It creates the idea of traumas by default and represents a decisive advance. A disorder caused by emptiness, therefore,

---

1 My italics.

but also by the excessive inner violence which has not been expressed. It does not express devastation due to excess that the lack can produce through the violent upheavals, rages and pains, both physical and psychic (but not differentiated in the baby) which have remained without an echo.

Winnicott thought patients had to be told that the fear they felt had already taken place and was "a fact hidden in the subconscious, not the repressed subconscious but part of the psyche close to the neurophysiological function". As far as my patients are concerned – those who have experienced these agonies at length but have not somehow "mentalized" their problems and have "chosen" the body – I do not think it necessary to tell them, but just to let them talk and repeat and repeat until they can develop a channel for distraction. If mentalization has been uncertain or poor, the after-shock of choice, so to speak, of early childhood traumas is the body, via the accidents, and above all pain, cathected as paradoxical mothering, protective and deadly but finally safe.

The repeated recital of the accident (itself an after-shock of previous traumas) represents an attempt to gain control of their life experience. But the clinic taught me that it was also an attempt to stage a violent primitive scene that had failed in its organising role. Whereas the screen memory is the result of condensation and displacement which masks the violence of the original fantasies, makes them manageable and operant and allows a rich fantasy life.

What do these states of lack and excess produce instead of what has not taken place? What becomes of the traumatic engrams created in this acute distress? In 1974, at about the same time as Winnicott – although I would not compare myself with him – I addressed two conferences where I talked about the engram. I described it at the time as a blank record, a non-figurative record (too many primary affects, not enough representations) which still leaves a mark and is capable of after-shock effects. If traumatic repetition is the consequence of a memory, I wondered what could be repeated by an engram which has none. More precisely, I said that a blank memory made up of too many unrepresentable stimuli is determined to repeat without much knowing what to repeat. I thought the subjects in question traumatophilic, using the old concept of traumatophilia, a predisposition or aptitude for trauma. Children who have known too much distress and have not been able to find representations, meanings or words for their distress may without knowing it repeat their traumatic state yet again later in pain. And they do not need a lesion for that.

TEMPORALITY, BEFORE AND AFTER SHOCK

Writers have intuitively taken up the idea of temporality marked by the need for repetition of both the after-shock sought by the psyche to find a meaning and create a psychic causality and a trauma seeming to be predestined.

Thus Henry James's hero Marcher thinks he destined for some great fate but does not know what it is. He often talks about it to a young woman who accompanies him in his expectation of and quest for the anticipated "Event". The young woman is suffering from a progressive disease and finally dies. Standing before her tomb, he suddenly realises that the event has already occurred: it is his relationship and his love for the young woman, and hers for him, of which he was unaware. "The escape would have been to love her ..." "He saw the Jungle of his life and saw the lurking Beast. He perceived it rise, huge and hideous, for the leap that was to settle him. He flung himself, face down, on the tomb."

In a short story entitled *Recall Mechanism* by Philip K. Dick who wrote science fiction suffused with psychoanalysis, a phobic vertigo sufferer searches desperately in his past and with analysts (who have to be on the ground floor!) for a reason for his terror of the void and fear of falling. The detailed exploration instituted by the analyst is no help to him because his screen memory is in the future. He suffers from a trauma that has not yet occurred and will take place at the end of the story: he falls from a plane. He had become *precog*, i.e. a "knower" of the future, after a major nuclear disaster which is perhaps the pre-shock that he was seeking. He knew his future and that was the cause of his phobia.

The traumatic engram fails to manufacture a screen memory. It is projected into the future, later. But what happens is a repetition of the trauma in one form or another: a scene relived in its hallucinatory dimension or in reality like Victor, or which freezes in pain or even renewed failure. The blind force of the repetition brushes the psyche aside. Pain can conceal this aspect of returning to the same thing because the mask of continuity and immovable repetition which it displays banishes the idea of repetitive attacks and disarms both the patient and the therapist. We must insert the active trauma which only aims to repeat itself into the sequence of forgotten traumas or, even better, help the patient to make it an after-shock, charged with meaning, and just a memory with the affects removed.

ÜBERDEUTLICH AND LATERAL CATHEXIS

It is very useful to provide a lightning conductor for one's own emotions by transferring one's attention to a secondary goal. Thus Freud said that he was going to the United States to meet a wild porcupine ... and address a few conferences. He dreaded his journey and also having to convince his American audience. The extraordinary thing is that he did actually see a porcupine in the Adirondacks! He also went to his conferences.

The idea that it is possible to defend oneself against any representation, memory or psychic structure by a lateral cathexis, i.e. close in spatial proximity rather than meaning, runs through Freud's work from beginning to end. Examples appear in manuscript K on hysteria, in the articles on screen memories (*Neurosis, psychosis and perversion*) and the split in the ego ("The fetish") and in "Constructions in analysis". The same defence mechanism can be seen when facing an unpleasant message from the repressed subconscious or a traumatic external perception. The stimulus is displaced to a neutral substitute structure, avoiding the one which would be painful. However, the neutral structure reflects the intense traumatic aspect of what is driven from the psyche (repressed or denied) by becoming *überdeutlich*, excessively clear or bright, as it is translated nowadays. This is the case with the yellow of Freiberg's dandelions or the brown bread in Freud's screen memory, the deformed face of Katarina's uncle and Lucy's strong smell of burnt pudding (in *Studies on hysteria*). In the case of amnesia that hides what is unpleasant, it is a substitute word that becomes bright. For example the word *exoriare*, which in the Latin verse misquoted by Freud's interlocutor comes just before *aliquis*, the forgotten word. P. Wilson quoted by Freud (1901) drew Freud's attention to the importance of the stress on the word *exoriare* which thus became *the imperceptible obvious*. It is impossible to know whether it is hiding what is important - or as Freud called it in Constructions "a piece of historical truth" - or whether it is the mark of what is important even if it is not its symbol.

The discourse of pain sufferers is monotonous at the beginning but sometimes suddenly becomes lively and almost joyful or even passionate. Coloured stains on a grey fabric. When they briefly occur, the patient stops suffering as though something is escaping the pressure of the pain. I have seen something similar with the phenomenon of brightness. For instance, a man who could only walk with crutches and proclaimed his pain throughout the session (quite realistically given the serious lesions he presented with) suddenly stopped to talk to us about philately and his stamp collection. Another patient with a hyperalgic disorder interrupted his complaints to tell us about his passion for old gold coins. He sometimes brought us some to admire. A third talked about "underground hunting" - badger baiting. I wondered when and why their speech became impassioned. It was always at a difficult time that a distraction took place to a small narcissistic enclave, a point of great satisfaction, a haven in the storm. Baubles no doubt, but anchor points chosen as a distraction from the pain.

They cannot really be described as "excessively clear". They are intense by their frequent occurrence, lifelines in an emergency and thus more insistent than bright. But they are part of the same mechanism, an energetic rejection of the displeasing and strong adherence to an old cathexis brought back to light.

Allowing these convulsions of life in the choking depths of the pain to live and blossom has often led to crucial associations. Whenever association has been possible, it has led to memories of childhood, screen memories from which the psychotherapy has been structured. Therein lies the secret of the rerouting and distraction. For instance, the gold coins, a narcissistic source of pride, had a raison d'être originating from a desolate childhood. The first small coin, not gold, received for services rendered had been carefully preserved like a fetish and, said the patient, was the starting point for what had changed his life.

These examples and those that follow show the mooring points or refuges which enable patients to forget their pain for a moment. They are ephemeral and the exigencies of the pain leave them little scope for development. The next two examples are different. I quote them to show how strange the pain clinic can be.

Monsieur P.'s story

An elderly man suffered from intense post-zosterian hemithoracic pain although he had had proper treatment. He said he was at the end of his tether and incapable of continuing to bear the sensations of burning and electric shock that tortured him day and night. I saw him regularly for some weeks. The situation deteriorated. The therapeutic arrangements carried out at my request by a highly competent neurological colleague had changed nothing. The pain invaded his mind and body and our relationship. The strong cathexes that had filled his life withdrew from both his psychic reality and his physical realisation capacity. But one had caught my attention: his passion for collecting the last vestiges of dialect in a particular part of the Ardèche. He had not spoken of this for some time. One day he said that he would not be returning and had decided to commit suicide, despite his strong religious convictions. The session proceeded in an atmosphere of extreme tension and in my case great anxiety. At the end of the session I shook his hand and instead of saying "au revoir" which I felt was too strong an incitement to return, I could only find one thing to say to him: The Ardèche ... leaving a sort of question mark. Then I followed him into the corridor which led either to the exit or to the administrative area. At the last minute he decided to make another appointment. In the sessions that followed it was in a different spirit, with some renewed vitality, that he began telling me again about the songs still sung by the old women of the Ardèche and his passion for the Oc languages, despite the ever-present pain. Had my intervention made him change his mind by evoking a cathexis so deeply rooted in him? I cannot say, but a corner had been turned.

Monsieur F.'s story

Monsieur F. came to see us due to complex vertebral pains. He was rather confused and interspersed his account with great bursts of infectious laughter. But the pains he described were intense, some of neuropathic origin, and were caused by lesions of the spinal cord. They required ad hoc treatment which he had not previously been given. We prescribed this and he was grateful. The other pains (nociceptive) responded to ordinary analgesic treatment. We had difficulty in describing this clinical picture to him because he was very confused, and also because of the strange atmosphere created by the laughter that erupted for no apparent reason. We could not stop ourselves laughing with him, although his recital of the violent pain he was suffering inclined us towards an empathy much more suited to its indisputable reality.

We learned that he had had not one but two accidents, both dramatic. The first preceded the second by a few years: Monsieur F. had had to stop on a motorway because of a tailback and a car travelling at high speed had hit him violently from behind and pushed him onto an obstruction. His car was wrecked and Monsieur F. suffered serious spinal injuries and multiple fractures. The second accident a few years later happened when Monsieur F. had not recovered from the first one: he had set out to go shopping in a town near his country home. It was winter; his car skidded on the icy surface and ended up down below the road. He had further spinal damage and various other injuries.

We followed up Monsieur F. regularly for years. It was one of the rare cases where my fellow therapist and I felt a need to discuss our patient regularly, as we were astonished by his great bursts of laughter that punctuated a narrative which was even more dramatic because Monsieur F. was clearly depressive and his pain did not improve. Trying not to burst out laughing and repressing with difficulty the loud guffaws that Monsieur F. provoked in us, we were prone to very bizarre feelings. Despite our comprehensive support, we felt guilty and experienced moments of unreality and even depersonalisation: how could we be moved by his pain and yet burst out laughing? And what to say about the depressive episode, so frequent among pain sufferers, that followed?

One fine day when Monsieur F. was much better (after being treated for several years at longer and longer intervals) he told me his secret, or at least the reason for his maniacal laughter. At the time of his second accident, when he was trapped in his car which was lying about two metres below the level of the road, he watched the following show: a second car skidded and came crashing down beside his and shortly afterwards a third car did the same and came to join them. In the ambulance taking our patient to hospital, he suddenly saw or rather had an insistent vision of something he could not escape: the three shattered cars broken down on the side of the road lying next to each other. An excessively clear vision, Freud would have said. And a repetitive phrase: "and one and two and three!" Monsieur F. collapsed into hysterical laughter which continued in hospital, to the great displeasure of the doctors.

On the day when he told me that, he did not laugh. He never laughed afterwards either. Monsieur F. had lost the memory of the excessively clear scene of his accident but had preserved the affect or motor response of the hysterical laughter in the ambulance and then in hospital which had astounded the doctors who kept saying: "Be quiet, there is nothing to laugh about". He did not remember that either.

The difficulty in these stories is the "Good God, it's obvious!" aspect which gives the impression of a key to be discovered or an archaeological treasure to be excavated. The patient I have just mentioned was followed up for years, at longer and longer intervals. He improved considerably in the course of time and his life became almost normal. His recent recovery of the forgotten reason for the hysterical laughter achieved nothing new except the final disappearance of the incomprehensible hilarity. My question on the subject of this exemplary case, though I could quote many others, is as follows: What was the function of the laughter, the unforgotten part of a traumatic memory whose essentials were forgotten or not functioning? What is the nature of the connection which that part established with us? It was important for that man to bring us his laughter and talk about his pain.

FROM COMPLAINT TO SELF-OBSERVATION: ROLE OF THE DOUBLE

To J. Lacan, it is through another person that the subject has access to an image of himself and this recognition occurs within language, the outside mediator.

In a short story called *A Descent into the Maelstrom*, Edgar Allan Poe narrates the adventures of two brothers dragged in their boat into a whirlpool that engulfs them. One of them observed that the lightest and most cylindrical objects were sucked into the chasm more slowly. He clung to a barrel and rose slowly back up the walls of the vortex while his brother was carried away with the boat.

This is how I have imagined the distraction which according to Freud allows one to be freed from the imprint of pain. Anyone who has heard the interminable sorrowful chant uttered by our pain patients at the beginning will also cling (as if to a barrel) to the small details that break free from the discourse. These are points that the regression has somehow highlighted, fixations about which the patient has much to say. Only language can bring them to life but it is often powerless to do so at the start. It is from them that the psychotherapy starts and develops. The patient sees himself otherwise than in pain, turns away from it and associates more freely. I will try to show the part played by the analyst in this difficult task.

I have talked about the psychic disposition of patients in pain, filled with great hope but also desperate and profoundly regressive. The initial treatment is monotonous and, as we have seen, characterised by endless repetition of the present suffering and the paradise lost. But usually this is soon replaced by dual work with the patient. The particular nature of our clinic means that this dual work is itself dual because it is done by both psychoanalysts (in our team P. Forestier and myself), obviously in different ways.

This dual work differs, for example, from what the Botellas described in the *French Journal of Psychoanalysis* (2001, No. 4) which alludes to very special moments in the analytical treatment which assume what they call "regredience" through which patient and analyst can approach thought transference phenomena.

We can never know another's pain; we can only know its words. These words change during the treatment and are good indicators of the patient's development. More than that, they are its living substance. The face-to-face situation used with our patients, because it is like a conversation, limits this kind of exchange but promotes others of a particular type. The recital of the complaints has to be changed to just a recital to access what I call the narrativity. At the beginning the regressive patient addresses an omnipotent parent from whom he demands a lot. The failure of the therapist to respond may be accompanied by disappointment (Laplanche's refusal) which aggravates the situation. The patient must progress from habitual repetitive self-description to a minimum of self-observation.

The image that has often come into my head during this progression is that of the imaginary friend used by Rosolato (1978). This is the friend that children between 4 and 5 years old often invent and with whom they have the relationship of a double. This double is the result of narcissistic self-worth projection and plays an important role because in this imaginary creation it is a defence against the loss of the object and therefore the anxiety of separation as well as castration. Rosolato talks about the dead child, the fantasy "A child is being killed" about which S. Leclaire wrote a book (1975), the theme and fantasy which is found so frequently among patients in pain but remains at the edge of consciousness and which the double can conjure up.

The double can take many forms. They range from an imaginary twin whose "troubling presence" can be persecution (Bion quoted by Ferro, 2000, p. 153), to forms offering the possibility of a different representation of oneself and therefore a richer imaginary identification game, an addition to the psyche. But the patient can change very quickly from one to the other.

The position of the psychoanalyst must be flexible and mobile, as in analysis but less neutral. The empathy he has to show towards patients necessarily contains moments of identification. The differences between sympathy and empathy are virtual and theoretical points. Faced with patients who are suffering and who experience moments of drama, I do not see how it is possible to avoid perpetual movement from one to the other. Empathy only exists through the authenticity of strong or violent shared emotions which have to be dismissed from the mind constantly, it is true. Of course it is not a matter of weeping with the patient. One must first suffer with the other person and then understand his suffering. And keep a variable distance, close enough to feel, far enough to continue to think. Too much sympathy aggravates the pain, not enough empathy removes the ability to influence it. It is sometimes necessary to react against these two feelings and not let oneself be invaded.

On the patient's part, we can observe that the start of release from the pain occurs at a moment of identification with the therapist, a moment of elation that can be compared with the jubilant assumption described by Lacan during the mirror stage. However brief these moments of exultation may be, they are important merely because they exist and are evidence of hope.

This dual work with the patient which is so important for the future of the therapy can emerge unexpectedly. Here is an example:

> This was a man who was really desperate, really monotonous and really difficult to tolerate. I was listening absent-mindedly when I heard him mention the Football World Cup which had been held the previous year, in 1998. My thoughts strayed to my memories of that time which had thrilled the whole of France. I spoke before coming out of from my torpor and heard myself say: "Yes, if Thuram had not scored two goals against Croatia, one on the right and one on the left – having never scored in his life – France would have been well and truly beaten!" I was shocked and surprised at this remark and wondered what I thought I was doing. My surprised patient said: "Well well! You are a doctor and are interested in football ... I was just thinking about Thuram myself!" We had become brothers and the dual work, genuine dual autoeroticism, was established.

It was a meeting of minds. It made me think of those *flare up* moments sometimes heard in the polyphonic music of New Orleans, when two musicians stopped improvising and in a brief moment of joyous complicity maintained an unplanned harmony before taking flight once again. My timely regression had produced an exchange which was quite unexpected but which I could see had an obvious function. The patient could begin talking to himself through me as if bouncing off me. A return to oneself by a detour through the other, as A. Green says (2002), was the first stage of the self-observation of the Ego which was previously impossible because it was buried under a repetitive self-description of the suffering. His pain facilitations were so deep that the Ego could not escape them and the impoverished language only described these compulsive facilitations. Therefore we operated differently, doubly autoerotic, homosexual and narcissistic, the three words being synonymous in this context.

In this furtive exchange, the patient's sudden metamorphosis astonished me. Just as a child can change from laughter to tears, so he had emerged from his customary difficult, slow state with an enthusiasm I would have not thought possible, the first sign of vitality. What he had seen in me was a mirror image of himself, but an image opposite to the one that the chronic pain had instilled: a joyful image. It was not yet self-observation, which allows expectation, self-criticism and thinking. But it was a start.

The double has many functions: although protective, they can easily become a persecution. Like pain, the double protects against the anxiety of annihilation and castration, but pain is firmly anchored whereas the double is mobile. The patient's animist regression drives him to divide himself between a part which clings to the narcissistic lifeline of pain, and another which identifies with the idealised images he projects onto the therapist. The relationship can then momentarily become a honeymoon. This fusion with the therapist is soothing for the patient, who forgets his pain, but a difference of opinion can soon evoke "the other one", the persecutor and therefore hated. The two valences of the pain sufferer's great ambivalence must be continually assessed.

The move from projection onto the double due to lack of representative containing possibilities – current at least - to internalisation – a discharge into the patient's psyche – is an important moment. Important and delicate, because the work of the analyst then moves away from a simple support operation, but cannot yet become truly interpretative. We do not know whether fanning the flames will produce an even stronger flame or put out the fire. We have to accept and promote the expression of the aggressive drives that are often masked by the face-to-face situation and incorporated in the atmosphere of cordiality and friendship that exists - and which risks drowning them in kindness. That would be a pity, because the externalisation which the projection involves is an attempt to escape the realm of pain. By enabling the patient to perceive and register them without endangering the rapport, he is given the opportunity to reincorporate them and achieve a meaning.

Having someone to listen passively is essential to the patient at the beginning. Listening forces the principle of reality and gives a secondary position to processes very close to the sensoriality of the pain, weighed down in the regression, and enables him to find different words and gain access to a more elevated, structured and elaborate level of language. It is rather like telling someone about a dream. Which is what patients do, sometimes to their great amazement (*Why am I telling you this?* they say), when they reach this stage. The listening naturally becomes more active then.

So the objective is to move from this dual function to self-observation. Freud says in *The Uncanny* that: "The idea of the double ... may, during the successive developments of the Ego, *acquire new contents*". These are the *mental consciousness* and *self-observation* which "allows the old representation of the double to acquire a new basis and many things are then attributed to it, mainly everything that appears in *criticism of oneself*"[1]. The move from dual functioning to self-observation, possibly critical, which represents the *new contents*, is accompanied by another extremely valuable valence, that of shared pleasure. The masochistic pleasure of complaint vanishes in favour of the pleasure of functioning as a pair.

ASSOCIATIVE NARRATIVE AND TRANSFERENCE

That the Ego, as Freud says in "Outline of a Scientific Psychology" watches itself at work is not inherent but something acquired. We have seen how this requires the effective presence of another and we recall the mothering

---

1 My italics.

function which allows thinking and pleasure in thinking, within the mother-child relationship. It is good for the therapist to let himself go and share the pleasure of functioning as a pair, knowing that it contains the danger of a pleasant but sterile fusion with the patient. He must therefore introduce a differentiation, a power of heterogeneity, which I would compare with Bion's maternal dreaming and its creative power. The psychoanalyst must be there, as a dispenser of the extraneous *into* the patient's psyche but *starting from* the patient's psyche. Fédida (personal conversation and 1985) spoke "of daytime residues, residues of life" and supported a very similar view: because the trauma sufferer destroys the language, and makes it impossible to form a daytime residue as an impression of life that has a language. These traumatised patients *cling* to the therapist (voice, face, look etc.) as if it is only from him that a dream in the night can be reconstructed; a dream that would be a language resource. I remarked to Fédida that – even more than this – the actual person of the analyst represents a daytime residue usable not only in the dream but also in the sometimes dreamlike reality established in a therapy session, even in the face-to-face situation.

The patient's regression that I spoke of earlier involves a return to the world of childhood but with one great difference: the child's dreaming. For example the world of the illusion of having created the transitional object – the imaginary friend – all this is founded in a creative world directed entirely towards the future. The child is an adult of the future. The patient in pain, even if regressive, remains an adult and his imagination is associated with lost illusions. The risk is great and it often happens that during our consultations we see a sudden defusion or deidentification emerging from the violence. It is like this: "You talk and talk but you are healthy and I am suffering! And it does not appear to interest you!" So we have to keep adjusting the distance from the patient, not too far and not too close, and retain some freedom of thought so that there can be a "Winnicottian" game with creative potential. In these cases it is good that there are two of us!

In one sense this sudden liberation from sadism is healthy because it allows the patient to escape from the painful masochism in which he is encased. Freud says that the sufferer is frozen in his anti-cathexis. In the case of pain, as we have seen, the masochistic position allows him to savour his pain in silence or sometimes in a loud voice. Whatever sense of guilt these patients may have is totally soaked up by the presence of pain. Because of this, the work that would be possible to mourn for the lost objects and the life of depression by means of guilty feelings disappears. It is the emergence of sadism during these attacks which represents a psychic event for the patient and a stage in the therapy: deidealisation of the two protagonists and emergence of guilt, which also has the advantage of being transferential. The object attacked has been the therapist, which has the merit of rehistoricizing the patient's actions by placing them within the sequence of similar memories. He can associate on scenes generally old and involving the parents. In any case, something has made its mark in the relationship with the therapist that he can use in his future interventions. The paradox of the situation is the need for fusion and defusion in turn to achieve individualization.

At this stage the initial discourse becomes different. A woman patient put it nicely to me one day: "The story of my life has replaced the story of my pain". This means that the patient has gained a freedom of cathexis which was impossible at the beginning because, as Freud said, the Ego impoverished by energy mobilised in the fight against pain is only capable of minimal functioning. The therapeutic word is governed by the method. The patient's discourse is shaped on the basis of an apparently trivial conversation which is not only not thwarted, but actually encouraged. Even better, a recital develops, still based on expressing the pain but more and more open. The patient's language then regains a polysemy which had dimmed or been totally lost due to the requirement for expression of the complaints. The patient tells a story instead of reliving it.

A relationship of trust is then established. The sufferer talks to himself as he talks to the psychoanalyst, through a dual eroticism greatly preferable to the initial painful autoeroticism. The patient sees us as a double and the differences between him and us are removed. He feels understood, which was not the case with his previous doctors. The regressive situation is favourable but certainly dangerous and we have to be aware that the problem of good and bad can soon return. Another danger is that the relationship can drag on and never achieve the desired objective, which is the exact opposite – autonomisation.

When the symptom does not take up so much of the conversation – which then becomes a conversation with the self bouncing off the therapist – the patient, without grasping the polysemic aspects of his speech, may use them without realising it. The importance of the work achieved can be measured by the affects that emerge. The patient has moved from the pleasure of expressing his complaints to the pleasure of the session and the pleasure of the relationship, rather like meeting a good friend. His recital has become much more narrative and rich. The most important thing is the interest he takes in his own psychic function, via the interest shown in him by the therapist, whose crucial role really does resemble that of a mother from whom one knows the importance of dreaming for the development of her child's mind.

Our purpose is to listen to the words and allow the patient to register them differently. It is a translation, but a translation which differs from that introduced by the pain and algetic neurosis dimension. In other words, firstly a detranslation, surely different from the one referred to by Laplanche (*French Journal of Psychoanalysis*, 1998, No. 3, about analysis) and therefore a look at the thought. No longer just thinking but looking at oneself thinking. Seeing oneself at work. Seeing oneself in the scene and observing oneself, which is what the traumatic memory does not allow. The traumatised patient has to relive his trauma. The patient has to be set on a path that will take him from the traumatic memory to the screen memory, which is now mobile, open and malleable and in which he sees himself.

The role of counter-transference is obviously fundamental in this enriching and diversifying feedback, which the patient can receive from the analyst and which has nothing to do with suggestion. The importance of looking at the situation face to face and the enormous demands from the patient who expects everything from us gives the transference a particular flavour. It is not a question of actually interpreting the transference but of using it constantly, which restores the patient to himself and his infantile neurosis.

The specific way in which our pain clinic is organised, with two minds at work, means that the patient sees the two analysts separately one after the other and develops a transferential situation with both. I did not foresee all the effects or the potential of this system. It has proved valuable for various reasons, but particularly because it can give the patient an opportunity to adopt different attitudes towards his two interlocutors and find material for development. The external object which each analyst forms increases the differentiation function and the possibilities of identification, especially if the primal identification movement was not of good quality when the ego was formed. In addition, the triangular relationship offered by the system, or rather the triplization, has an effect even if it is directed towards a personality little structured by the Oedipus complex. Firstly, it shows that the other person, the one not participating in the dual scene, is not destroyed, thanks to the assumed complicity between the therapists, and for that reason too is not a persecutor. Secondly, as was the case with the example below, the patient can communicate more flexibly with his internal images which it is less necessary to control, protect or defend against.

The fact that we do not often discuss our patients certainly favours free expression of the two transferences. What generally happens, at least initially, is a division between bad and good, one of us being the good guy and the other the bad guy, usually alternately. The fact that there is always at least one good guy allows the relationship to remain sound and easier to maintain. In the example which follows, illustrating the benefits of our twin consultations, the division is different and the maternal and paternal functions projected onto us by the patient are different.

This patient appeared unconquerable because he was frozen in his pain, his language, his problems and in time. He suddenly began to progress and change following a discussion between P. Forestier and myself. We realised that despite the same blanket words that he used to us both, we had two different patients.

Monsieur G.

Monsieur G. was a large man weighing 130 kg. He had had his accident a few years before coming to see us. A terrible accident, he told us: "I was stabbed in the back by a fork". It turned out to be one of the two forks of a large lift truck rather than an agricultural implement. A piece of steel one and a half centimetres thick by twelve wide went very deeply into his back and left him transfixed and unable to move. It was evening and the site was deserted. Fortunately a late worker heard his cries and called the emergency services. The serious damage caused lesions to the various tissues of the spinal column and brought him much pain, particularly very intense neuropathic pain. He tried to go back to work without success and had to give up his job. Monsieur G. was registered disabled by social security. He missed his job and his friends. He felt alone and lived "sadly" with his mother. Before he had never stopped all day, now he felt useless. And he suffered day and night.

- "It hurts, it hurts a lot, it hurts here, where I was stabbed, and it goes down there and then further down where it really hurts." He went over his whole body, his leg, shoulder and the other side from top to bottom, not to mention the neck and the ears that whistled and "hurt, hurt a lot". It was worse at night. Nightmares forced him to relive his accident and during the day he had visions of it. He hated it.

For months and months Monsieur G. repeated the same words down to the last comma at every session, first to me and then to my colleague, and there was no change in his pain either. The stereotypical nature of his discourse irritated us but not his complaints, which we felt to me immense and well beyond the simple expression of his physical pain, which was certainly very intense. It showed us the wreck of a life. But only the body was mentioned. We listened attentively on several levels, based on an empathy that made me think of maternal preoccupation or dreaming. It was not a passive basis. We expressed ourselves, offering what might be accepted as anti-cathexes or falling silent, which demonstrated our interest. And one day we realised during one of our discussions about him - which were infrequent because we wanted to retain our own specific methods - that Monsieur G. was beginning to differentiate between us.

I had the impression that he was making me play a rather maternal role. From the depths of his regression, he talked to me about his chronic green or yellow "runs", his gall bladder and his digestive problems. He had no appetite. He complained of losing weight, which was not obvious to me but I understood that he wanted me to be concerned about it, as his mother had once been. It is true that a baby's digestion and weight gain are the mother's concerns. He regaled me unreservedly with his feeding and digestive symptoms. At that time his complaints were more important to him than his symptoms. He expected understanding rather than healing from his mother.

To my colleague he expounded the details of a rather mechanistic theory he had formulated. The lift truck fork had made a big hole in his loins. It was a void that had to be filled. The flesh had gone back up, the leg too, which made him shorter and caused an imbalance to his whole hemicorpus, spinal column, bone structure, other leg, arms and neck. This explained the generalised pain and also the damage caused to his liver, an after-effect of the shock of the fork.

Monsieur G. therefore reserved for my colleague a technical standpoint which was an aetiology, demonstrating an attempt to regain control over the pain in his limbs, which are organs of activity, by explaining the mechanism; as a small boy discusses the mysteries and theories of the world with his father. I was made the recipient of his anxiety about a digestive disorder he considered serious and progressive. The consequence of the aetiology. He was able to project images onto us, more or less maternal for me and paternal for my colleague, through the different qualities of our presence. The repetitive complaints continued, but Monsieur G.'s psyche could begin to decathect by working things through in his mind.

Conclusion

Narrativity and Work of the Analyst

The structure is developed in the actual process of emergence of the words. There is no contract, no rule to be observed: "Say what comes into your head". The analyst's attention drifts around in different ways and can and must be caught from time to time by the conversation. But his third ear, the analytical one, must remain vigilant.

Consensus and compliance are soon built up. The patient accepts our position and subscribes to it and his words soon begin to resemble what free association produces. What Freud invented, the singularity of the analysis session with the patient talking freely and the analyst, listening without replying, must represent something profoundly human, probably inherited from the parent-child situation. This is what allows the patient to watch his thoughts emerging from the narration when they detach themselves from it.

How should we assess our work with our pain patients? Thinking about this after so many years, I realise that the greatest change in them is in their language. The sovereignty of pain over their ego is initially manifested in the implosion of language, overwhelmed because I have called up the need for complaint and the reality of the presence of the pain. In this system the representative activity is constantly upset by perception of the pain, a true foreign body. The impoverished ego talks to itself about its downfall, as in depressive patients, but its internal narrative does not have fluency and is criss-crossed by all that the pain corrodes and demands.

When patients start improving, this is reflected in the less frequent mention of pain in their speech and above all because they talk better and differently. They are no longer in a closed circuit without outlets but in a shared system in which identification is possible without being alienating, therefore open to the world. The narrative exchange, like the pain and the hyperactivity, contains both a stimulus and the discharge of that stimulus. This is precisely because it is an exchange, like the one that once took place with the parents.

An even more archaic exchange is the one represented by the encounter between the mother's dreaming and the baby. Maternal dreaming – that singular phenomenon by which the psyche is developed and humanity is transmitted.

> "The baby seeing the mother dreaming identifies with her and the pleasure she has in dreaming." (Hochmann, 2001)

Can this be compared with the many small psychic incidents that enter the analyst's mind as he works and is it possible to say that their resonance in him and his responses have effects similar to those of maternal dreaming?

This question can be broadened and extended to psychoanalysis itself. What is effective in psychoanalysis? What do the structure, configuration, technique etc. produce? Above all, dealing with what has been repressed as part of the transference between a patient who associates and an analyst. What is being analysed is the resistance. That which is interpreted and constructed by the analyst is done here and now. The translation work which emerges is that of the actual words spoken to the analyst now. Psychoanalysis is not archaeology, not the work of the historian and not a discussion with the patient illuminated by psychoanalytical theory.

Having said that, the analyst's theoretical system and internalised knowledge have a part to play. Here it is clear that the Anglo-Saxons, for example, use a different theoretical tool from non-Kleinian French analysts. Belief in a theory can give rise to belief in what is effective in the treatment.

In the light of some aspects of narrativist thought (Schafer, A. Ferro), which challenge this point, the question arises as to whether the narration itself might have a therapeutic effect through the reorganisation it generates. I quote from J. Hochmann:

> "Schafer thinks that the object of psychoanalysis and its efficacy lie not in the discovery of a historical or fantasised reality but in the construction, by close collaboration between the analyst and his patient, of a narrative which gives meaning to the past." (*ibid.*)

The object of the analysis in Schafer's eyes is therefore "to give the patient, the co-narrator of his history, a greater narrative flexibility, help him deconstruct histories to which he clings, sometimes defensively, to allow new forms to emerge..."

Deconstruct-reconstruct or detranslate-retranslate – the two processes are very similar. They define an object and not the manner of achieving it. As to the manner, I repeat what I said earlier. But I like and am impressed by the expression "co-narrator of his narrative" because this is how I see my pain patients who, I emphasise again, are not undergoing an analytical process. They are in the process of psychotherapy with an analyst. This psychotherapy aims to redistribute the energy immobilised by the pain and tear a regressive but living psychic problem from it which it has both masked and aggravated; to disentangle it. The pain psychizes and becomes more like suffering through grief and depression, a mental pain. Separation anxiety, distress and also aggression then appear and the process is more like the habitual work of the psychoanalyst. It is possible to measure the active part played by him in this development, this process of emergence which is both the cause and the consequence of the implosion of the narrative.

J. Hochmann is a reader of Ricoeur, particularly *Time and Narrative* (Seuil 1983), and takes his inspiration from the three stages developed by him (prefiguration, configuration and refiguration). He attempts to apply them to the qualities of maternal dreaming, as narrative, narrative addressed to a third party and source of pleasure obtained from flexible handling of the language exchange, attentive to the transferential fluctuations.

- *Prefiguration* is what has happened, the event; for example: two chariots pass each other on the Thebes road, an altercation, one of the drivers, Oedipus, kills the other, Laios, etc.
- *Configuration* is its narrative. An affair and involvement of a causality: the oracles, father, mother etc. "one" talks of.

- *Refiguration* is the history that ensues, narrated to someone, the Oedipus Myth.

These three stages match the development of our patients' words. Under the shock of the pain trauma and probably influenced by the "interrogatory" attitude of their previous medical experience, their narrative sees itself at the beginning as a photograph of what has happened. But if the circumstances are right, they open up more and more and end by associating more freely, though still locked into the need for repetition associated with trauma. It is the involvement of the analyst, even if he is often reserved (but not always, as we have seen with the Thuram episode!) that is the foundation for what becomes co-narration. This involvement leads the patient, who is both the narrator and the main hero, to have a different view of his own history, unintentionally reflected, as if by a mirror, by the other person, in this case the analyst.

This happens in Proust. I quote from Bernard Raffalli, who wrote a brilliant and astute preface to an edition of *Remembrance of Things Past*:

> "This edifice rests on a person, both narrator and main hero, whom Proust describes in the first person "I" or the third person "Marcel". This gives the narrative its "mobility and its development through the diversity of his view". The Narrator is and is not Proust, of whom Raffalli says that he had "that breathtaking gift of seeing himself in others". Adding these apt words: "The narrator becomes the author to talk about a narrator who would become an author".

This distancing between the patient who says I and the one who contemplates himself in the eyes of the other in his own language emanation sets him apart from his painful affects and perceptions, removes him from his algetic neurosis and helps to restore him to his former affective world. The first steps towards emancipation from pain.

This language transformation work accomplished by the patient as his situation develops is naturally only possible by other work, that of the psychoanalyst. The new language now expresses fantasies as well as the complaints, which will gradually diminish. The patient has become consolable and addresses his mother. The image is that of the *Mater Dolorosa* gathering her child to her which as time passes becomes, more banally, "Mummy, it hurts". Onto this is then superimposed another harsher image addressed to the father, which is a reproach: "Father, can't you see I'm burning?" like the child in the first dream presented by Freud in *The Interpretation of Dreams*. This aspect has to be dealt with further.

This book is a testimony based on long experience. I want it to reflect the passionate enthusiasm of the analysts who have worked with me and, of course, my own. I would like others to follow my lead, because this is a vast unexplored field. Psychoanalysis, which is questioning its own future, must make its voice heard here, as Sigmund Freud did in Vienna more than a century ago, listening to patients talking about their pain.

Appendix

THE PAIN CLINIC AT LYON NEUROLOGICAL HOSPITAL

Some years ago I worked regularly twice a week in the rheumatology department under Professor Vignon and questioned the impact my presence was having in the department. I had been called in not so much to resolve the patients' pain problems as to show the doctors how not to reject the "incurables" – the lumbalgic patients called psychogenic. Rheumatism is painful and afterwards I had an opportunity to see many other forms of physical suffering. I was reasonably satisfied with the work I had done with the doctors. They seemed liberated and more at ease and had acquired the kind of expertise which incorporated proposals for therapy and treatment which were systemized and therefore reassuring.

But I had many questions for myself about the results achieved with the patients concerned. I might have succeeded with the doctors but I appeared to have failed with the patients. Basically, I had transferred the doctors' problem to myself and the patients seemed to me to be suffering just as much when they left as when they were hospitalised. My involvement as a kind of mediator between the protagonists had reassured the doctors but not relieved the patients.

It was then that a student completing her studies (Barruel) who was very interested in my work with the chronic pain sufferers had the idea of writing her thesis on the subject. She sent a very simple questionnaire to thirty-four recently hospitalised patients, all suffering from post-traumatic pain.

Four questions were asked.

1. Are you still in pain?
2. Are you back at work?
3. Since when?
4. Are you still having treatment?

Seventeen patients replied. In answer to the first question, sixteen said they were in just as much pain and only one felt cured. But on the second question, nine said they had returned to work against eight who were still not working. The answers to the third and fourth questions offered nothing of great significance. The questionnaire made me more optimistic: it seemed to open up the possibility of psychotherapy for chronic pain sufferers, particularly as the patients - nearly all victims of work-related accidents - had not worked for some time, the majority for several months and in two cases several years (three and five years), and had now resumed their jobs. Perhaps they had gone into hospital at a time when they felt recovery was possible.

In any case it was easier for the patients to say that they had gone back to work than to "admit" that they were in less pain. I use the word admit deliberately because our experience at the pain clinic has shown that it is the one often used by patients who are improving, as if it is wrong to stop feeling the pain or they have some difficulty in abandoning the painful situation that has developed. The results of the questionnaire reassured me about the possibility of mobilising patients who seemed to be trapped in their world of pain. I then decided to set up a facility to treat patients in chronic pain in the medical psychology department at Lyon

Neurological Hospital (Professor J. Guyotat, then Professor J. Dalery).

THE TOOL

A tool had to be worked out. The rheumatology department at the general hospital where I had gained my experience was very well organised: very interested doctors, caring nurses who had become experts in the course of time, a large team of highly motivated physiotherapists with very modern equipment, facilitating the psychic regression which the hospitalisation itself allows, by physical "abandonment" (their word) promoted by massage, various treatments and exercises in the warm water pool. The patients, as well as the doctors, felt reassured by the very technical but also very maternal environment provided for them.

But in my department at the neurological hospital I was alone. I had an idea that I would establish a pain clinic of a very particular type, run entirely by psychiatrists who should preferably be psychoanalysts. I had a free hand because our department was in a teaching hospital and, more importantly, a research hospital. The department head, deputy head, head clinician, psychologists, house doctors and junior doctors were all analysts or working in analysis. I had no difficulty in setting up a system that I intended should be simple and adaptable to extend the experience I had begun to acquire at the general hospital and to do that I conceived the idea of working in tandem with a colleague and friend who was himself an analyst.

I describe it not as an example but to show both the problems and the potential of pain treatment, potential and problems which caused me to hesitate. An odd occurrence removed any lingering doubts. A patient who was to be the last at the clinic presided over before the specific pain clinic opened dubbed himself number zero (therefore before number one, which he told me was the custom in the press) at the new clinic. I shall never know how he had heard it would be opening. A road accident had caused some sort of tear in his thigh and he suffered from deafferentation pain: intense electrical discharges all along the nerve that had been injured, from thigh to knee. His condition had improved after suitable treatment and he was reassured by our conversations. At our last meeting he confided an astonishing thing to me: during sex the sensation of orgasm followed the path of the pain, which was then transformed into pleasure. I decided that it was exciting that pain could conceal such mysteries. Our relationship was an easy one and our exchanges were even pleasant, quite different from what I might have expected in the light of the intensity of his ingrained, obdurate pains, and the patient said he felt better.

Strangely, it was a joke attributed to Alexandre Dumas that enabled me to find a system that could be effective: "The chains of marriage are so heavy", he said, "that it sometimes takes three to support them". I established two-man consultations to support the chains of pain which are also very heavy. What followed showed how effective and convenient that arrangement was. Each patient would be seen first by me and then by my colleague at each consultation, each conversation lasting half an hour.

Our selection criterion is simple: we welcome to the clinic any patient who claims to be suffering. Some present with severe organic disorders (neurogenic and post-zosterian pain, phantom sensations, hemithalamic syndromes), while others would be labelled differently as hypochondriac hysterics or post-traumatic neurotics. However the majority suffer from a combination of pathologies because the clinical pictures are often confused and the somatic and the psychic overflow into each other. We therefore decided to leave it to the somaticians to come up with a precise and rigorous diagnosis, allowing us to devote our attention to the problems associated with the expression, experience and cathexis of the pain felt, our goal being integration of those problems into the psyche. Nearly all our patients are people who have been let down by medicine for one reason or another and have long been suffering. They may have protested. We are often their last hope.

As I said before, the patients' imagination is expressed in associative structuring, aetiological inventions and quite arbitrary connections and logic which confound the conventional doctor and sometimes irritate him. The patient may then feel misunderstood and this marks the start of the break in the therapeutic alliance. The medical environment is no longer reassuring for either of them; there is a divergence and at relational level an ambivalence, a shared disappointment. This is particularly true when the doctor has failed, which is mainly seen with somatic patients with resistant disorders but also in patients with psychogenic pain; in short, with nearly all the patients we see at our clinic.

THE PRINCIPLES

The idea is therefore to promote what is usually discouraged so as to offer:

- The widest possible scope for expression of the imagination;
- But also a structure that allows some process of elaboration.

When pain invades a subject's whole life, some common parameters appear which we have to take into account.

The first of these is regression: regression to the time of childhood and even further to the archetypal and original, to the memory of the primal distressed state (*Hilflosigkeit*) that every human new-born baby has known.

This regression is naturally accompanied by dependence that recalls the baby's dependence on its mother and links the patient to his doctor, sometimes like a heavy weight. Added to this is a feeling of impotence experienced as depressive.

The eager and insistent demand for care, also a heavy weight, belongs in the same context and goes along with the need to complain.

Last but not least, the ambivalence of our patients associated with the other three parameters demands very great powers of adaptation and handling of distance because the object, that is ourselves, is invested with good or bad qualities according to the circumstances.

To meet these difficult demands, our consultations are two-man. At each session the patient is seen first by a psychiatrist/psychoanalyst for half an hour and immediately afterwards by a colleague who is also a psychiatrist/psychoanalyst, again for half an hour. The roles and functions of the two doctors are very different, very precise and defined in detail but are not revealed to the patient unless he asks (which has never yet happened).

THE PROCEDURE

First consultation

This is in the form of a nondirective conversation which is mainly aimed at allowing the patient's discourse to develop. What appears then is not the distress or the pain but the discourse about the distress or pain. The important points are underlined automatically by surprising associations, strange causalities, hesitations and especially repetitions. We can then perceive how the psyche has registered and integrated the pain and associated trauma, and the pathogenic power they have retained.

These conversations highlight the points referred to above: the intensity of the demands, the desire for self-expression, the tendency towards dependence etc. All this promotes the development of a rapport. Unlike Scotland Yard in the old days, where a poster on the wall indicated or warned that "Anything you say will be used against you", the patient realises that here it is the opposite: everything will be used "for" him.

But the pain, loss of bodily integrity, goodbye to or renunciation of the physical and even intellectual capabilities of the past before the pain and the restrictions it imposes give birth to a new self-image and new narcissistic cathexes. The patient sets some store by the pain and the help he is asking for. Like a small child suffering, he wants to be loved and cared for. This aspect is also a mark of a good rapport but we can see the danger in it: hope disappointed and expectation of improvement cheated may plunge the patient into an ambivalent and then aggressive attitude.

The therapist is then in a more difficult situation and must adapt, be less reserved and open up a little. This is not sufficient in itself to maintain an adequate rapport, which is why there is a second therapeutic focus of a completely different type. It is the play between the two which allows the ambivalence to be expressed and handled. For example, one of us can be the good guy and the other the bad guy and both therapists have to adapt.

Second consultation

The second part of the consultation is much more "medical". It focuses on the pain symptoms from a wholly physical standpoint and includes questionnaires.

The first is a conventional pain questionnaire similar to those used in other clinics or centres. Its purpose is to enable the patient to describe the nature of his pain in detail:

- Its location: two human silhouettes are shown to patients. They are asked to draw the path of the pain and indicate the places where it is most acute;
- Its nature: they are asked to choose from a selection of words or phrases the one that best describes it (hammering, shooting, churning, tearing, burning pain etc., irritating, exhausting, troubling, distressing, unbearable, agonising, gnawing, causing suicidal feelings etc.);
- Its timing: the patient indicates on a table dividing the day (morning, afternoon, evening, night...) how the pain changes over the nycthemeron, when it appears, when it improves or disappears, whether it is continuous, whether it goes away at night and allows sleep etc.;

- The methods the patients use to fight it: medication, rest, cold, heat, massage or other techniques;
- The circumstances or conditions that aggravate it: fatigue, stress postures...;
- Its intensity: this is assessed by the patients themselves by ticking a horizontal scale with the zero at the right and the maximum on the left to prevent a reflex response from habit (the patient has to think more about his response);
- Its consequences and effect on the patient's sleep, social and sex life and professional and leisure activities.

The second questionnaire is Kincannon's Minimult (MMPI).

It is a personality test. Seventy-one general questions are asked; the test has three validity scales and nine others evaluate aspects of personality and character (anxiety, depression, hysteria, paranoia, schizophrenia, somatisation etc.). The results are analysed by computer.

The second psychoanalyst is also responsible for prescribing medication, looking after the administrative records and maintaining links with the attending physicians.

THE DEVELOPMENT

The first part is therefore fully open to the spontaneous narrative of the patients and thus to the psyche. The second is closer to a somatic concern. I set up this system without really thinking that it represented the opposite of what normally happens medically, when "psychogenic" diagnoses are often made by elimination: we cannot find anything so it must be psychological, and then the patient is sent to a psychiatrist. My colleague and friend P. Forestier who kindly agreed to take over responsibility for the second part remarked to me that in addition to opening up a new world to patients by flattering their narcissism, which was certainly in need of it, this reverse order also had a highly stimulating effect on their generally rather depressive economy.

After the first session the patients are normally very surprised because "nothing much has been done to them", but they readily agree to return. The treatment we can offer them is set up and the long psychotherapy begins. I have to say that the roles of the two doctors which are strongly differentiated at the beginning lose some but not all of their specific characteristics and both then operate freely.

Our first concern is to prevent our patients repeating with us what has happened with their doctors, sometimes many of them, who have failed to resolve their pain problem. We know that the more disappointed they are, the more demanding they are. We know their regression, we know their distress, their feelings of impotence, their abandonment fantasies and their ambivalence, simultaneously guilty and aggressive. We offer them a different and seemingly non medical attitude, which surprises them but in which they join. Initially at least, we refuse to feel a fanatical desire to cure them – a dangerous *furor sanandi* – because it would be accompanied by an inability to tolerate the slightest failure. We replace it with an equally fanatical desire to create the link and maintain the rapport at all costs.

There was a risk: What I was offering to patients suffering physically was therapy on and through words. A talking cure. The words still had to come out. My experience with lumbalgics and hypochondriacs had shown me not only that they were capable of uttering words, discourse and even narrative (in different registers it is true), but also that they were keen to do so.

Our work lasted for about twenty years. We never needed to change the principle, which proved ideal for our purposes. The following pages show how it developed and particularly the unexpected consequences of there being two of us, both in the quality of the narrative and the transferential aspect.

I believe I felt guilty about this transferential aspect. The patients had come to cure their pain, not for psychotherapy. I used a hypocritical ruse to introduce them to a process they did not want and had not cathected by previous thought. I had told my colleagues that we must answer all questions or requests for information about our treatment methods. There were practically none.

CLINICAL EXAMPLE

The clinical example below illustrates how the pain clinic at Lyon Neurological Hospital operated and shows in particular how the two-man system can facilitate the emergence in the patient of some kind of psychic event which opens up the elaborative potential more easily.

She was a patient speaking poor French who was followed up by our second team consisting of Dr. Marcombes and Dr. Forestier. The first was run by Dr. Forestier and myself.

Report by Dr. Marcombes

> Mme E. was referred to us for a polyalgetic syndrome which was intensifying and had lasted three years. She had consulted numerous doctors for scapular, cervico-brachial lumbar, then abdominal and finally cephalic pain. When she came, her body was painful from her head to her knees. The pains were located in the joints and muscles. We were brought in by an algologist who, after several months of specialist care, was in difficulty due to the woman's desperation and demands that her distress be recognised. She had stopped work more than two years earlier and was in dispute with the health insurance organisation involved. She came to contest the decision of the medical examiner who required her to return to work, refusing to give a disability decision that was not well supported by medical opinion.
>
> This 45 year old woman was an immigrant. She was born in Italy and lived there until the age of twenty.
>
> At our first meeting she cried and listed all the painful parts of her body, with suffering that was pathetic to see. Her discourse was an imagined evocation. From the first conversation her physical representations were associated

with a narrative of events in which violence, brutal scenes and affective losses could be read.

> "It began in a butcher's shop where I worked, with the cold of the freezer, my shoulder stiffened ... I was 35 ... A few years later I decided to leave, I was tired, my stomach and back hurt... butchery is hard... I was six weeks pregnant but did not know, I lost my rights ... I had had a curettage previously...My stomach swelled: twins, one died in the uterus, I had my last daughter, my fourth child ..."

She interrupted her narrative, sobbed, and resumed:

> "The pain beats in my head, there is a hammer, a bombardment in my ears ... At 35 I was trapped on a staircase by a boy with a knife in my back. We were overheard and I managed to escape... My fingers, these two – she indicated the third and fourth – they have been dead... my knees, I can no longer climb up and down ... my muscles, they hurt."

When we asked her to localise the pain on the human silhouettes – asexual – on our questionnaire, she would not do so at first and wondered if it was a woman. Then she stopped drawing: Are these the buttocks? (They are clearly shown). In contrast, she only seemed to see the many black marks on the paper. She became animated when she described the algetic physical sensations which she detailed for each part of the body.

During the first months of the treatment Madame E. improved and enriched her tragic narrative. The death of her parents in particular (her father of a cerebral haemorrhage and her mother of cancer of the colon a year later to the day) was systematically associated by her with uterus surgery a year before the event that could be identified with her problems:

> "The day my father died, I bled ... No, I think it was my mother... Her intestines had burst, the surgeon made a mistake; there are two intestines and he took the wrong one... She suffered terribly and my illness began just afterwards ..."

For about 18 months her pains persisted and even worsened, while gradually losing their polyalgetic character (the complaints of pain were then only about one shoulder or the stomach and back combined). Her depression also became more intense. She remained in dispute with the insurance company after a disability decision by the health insurance organisation and persisted with her claim against the doctors (particularly the surgeon who had operated on her mother).

Losing a child (we learned that one brother and one sister – out of twelve siblings – had died of disease at between two and three years old), losing a parent, being sexually abused: these scenes were detailed innumerable times in different versions by her narrative of events, memories and dreams. But we gradually noticed a change and some elaborative movement (for example in the way she talked about her body, venturing imaginary connections between the stomach and the shoulder... between the pain in her side and pregnancy... between the surgery undergone by herself and her mother...)

One moment appeared particularly important to us, two years after the start of her treatment. We had noticed that she was reticent about talking in the presence of the first practitioner but talked freely to the second. On an occasion when the first interlocutor was absent, she clearly expressed her ambivalence towards him precisely in terms of fear. She alluded to the couch in his consulting room and then to a scene of rape by her brother when she was a child (what she had never been able to mention – even to herself – had come back to her a few weeks earlier in an anxiety dream).

Report by Dr. Forestier

What must be considered a true confession by this patient represented a turning point in our treatment. It was the start of a new discourse that raised questions previously hidden by her incessant and insistent talking about the pain phenomena. These new questions related to her being, her female being. After that she began talking about her relationship with her husband, who did not understand her and had never really "considered" her:

"People who go to see psychiatrists are mad," he told her. She then asked herself about her own "madness". In fact her most fundamental question emerged, the question of being a woman and her relations with the opposite sex. We were then part of a more precise elaboration; a sort of hystericization and a new process of development of the unconscious began. The signifier 'mal' then acquired another aspect with its ambiguous meaning: male – in the stomach. It was sex that was at the top of the agenda and represented the real and original trauma, by reference to Freud's teaching.

We chose this case from the many that we see at our clinic because it is typical in a number of ways:

- It illustrates the factors described above by Gabriel Burloux which can be found in all patients called chronic pain sufferers: dependence, ambivalence and temperospatial regression as effects of chronic pain. The great scope for imagination gives the discourse of these patients a very particular tone and with this one in particular the confusion about either the dates or the physical manifestations. The many traumatic events since her childhood which had punctuated her lengthy, plaintive discourse like a sequence up to that seemingly minor accident categorised her as a chronic pain patient;
- The original two-man system, as we like to call it, together with psychoanalytical orientation, favoured the emergence of a change of subjective position. The trauma came from the Other and it all happened as though the subject could only suffer what happened to her. After the time that we call her confession, the subject took her share of responsibility in the sense that she was responsible for what she said and from then on she could start working on the part of her psyche that had "escaped" her;
- The specific treatment at our clinic showed the function of the pain. It was a reminder of the early Freud in his *Studies on Hysteria* where physical pain takes the place of mental pain. The pain expressed in the body that could not be expressed otherwise, in the form of either anxiety or depression. The psyche was actually

bypassed for lack of possible elaboration or even representation during the trauma. The need for mourning associated with the sequence of losses allowed this psychic elaboration. The long period of the first part of the treatment which extended over two years was necessary both to accept the painful complaints and to allow the patient to put her history in order: to order the sequence of events and give a meaning to the "different traumas" by replacing them in her history;

- The importance of the transferential relationship. We could not speak of transference in the strict sense of the word because of the particular structure we offered. In the first stage of the treatment the therapist was a "party" to the words spoken to him. The patient was actually addressing her complaints of pain to the "pain specialist" at the general hospital. These complaints had to be accepted without losing sight of the aims of the therapy we offer to these patients, which is psychic elaboration to allow integration of the pain within the psyche. Note that it was due to the absence of one of the two therapists, the one who was first to accept it, that the confession was made and proved a real turning point in the treatment and the effect on the patient just mentioned.

Certainly this involves a genuine psychoanalytical process in the sense of a conventional cure, and the reference to the psychoanalysis by the therapists allows this development in those patients who are truly "fixed" in this pain, cathecting it to a maximum and therefore being unable to cathect anything else. The process gradually produces a reduction in the cathexis of the pain and promotes new cathexes. This work is still going on and the road is still long for this particular patient before she can really extricate herself from everything that has shackled her up to now and can envisage a new "construction". The latest encounters have indicated the importance in this subject of the scopic drive, which is declined in the same way as grammar: to see, be seen, see oneself... and have given us a new direction for the process.

Chronic pain patients represent a new category defined by modern medicine, with a series of common features which we have mentioned above. On this basis it is both a trauma clinic and a mourning clinic associated with losses. But psychoanalysis teaches us that it is a clinic of the individual where each case must be examined separately. It is this dimension of an encounter which is new every time and renewed every time which maintains our enthusiasm for treating these very difficult patients. It is this enthusiasm that we want to communicate.

BIBLIOGRAPHY

ANTELME J. (1996), *The Human Species*, Paris, Gallimard.
ANZIEU D. (1975), *Freud's Self-Analysis*, vol. 1 and 2, Paris, Puf.
AUBERT A. (1966), *Pain*, Paris, Puf.
AULAGNIER P. (1975), *The Violence of Interpretation: From Pictogram to Statement*, Paris, Puf.
BARRUEL E. (1981), "Psychogenic Rachialgia", Thesis, Lyon 2.
BAYLE G. (1996), "Splits", *Paris Psychoanalytical Society Bulletin*, No. 39
BEETSCHEN A. (1989), "The stimulus of loss", *New Journal of Psychoanalysis*, No. 39
BEETSCHEN A. (2002), Proceedings of the French-language Psychoanalysists Conference, *Paris Psychoanalytical Society Bulletin,* "Accomplishment and Achievement".
BERGERET J. (1972), *Digest of Pathological Psychology*, Masson.
BERGERET J. (1974), *The Normal and Pathological Personality*, Dunod revised edition 1996.
BERGERET J. (1984), *Fundamental Violence*, Paris, Dunod.
BERGERET J. (1985), *Freud, Violence and Depression*, Puf.
BERGERET J. (1999), *Narcissistic Eroticism*, Paris, Dunod.
BOTELLA C. & S. (1984), "Unconscious homosexuality and the dynamic of the double in the analysis session", *French Journal of Psychoanalysis*, No. 3.
BOTELLA C. & S. (2001), in *French Journal of Psychoanalysis*, No. 4.
BRADBURY R. (1940), *Martian Chronicles*, Paris, Gallimard, Coll. Folio, 2001.
BRETTE F. (1982), "From trauma and hysteria to recovery" in J. Guillaumin *Fifteen Psychoanalytical Studies over time*, Toulouse, Private, pp. 41-54
BRETTE F. (1985), "Argument for a certain hysteria", *French Journal of Psychoanalysis*, No. 1.
BRETTE F. (1986), "From somatic compliance to depressive compliance", *French Journal of Psychoanalysis*, No. 3.
BRETTE F. (2000), "Hysteria and trauma", *French Journal of Psychoanalysis* Monograph
BURLOUX G. (1974), "The amnesiac trace", Conference at Lyon Neurological Hospital.
CANDALIS-HUISMAN D. (1999), "The distressed state of the newborn", in *Distressed States* (ed. J. André, C. Chabert), Paris, Puf.

CASTORIADIS-AULAGNIER P. (1975), *The Violence of Interpretation*, Paris, Puf.
CHABERT C. (1999), "Introduction" in *Distressed States* (ed. J. André, C. Chabert), Paris, Puf.
COSNIER J. (1977), "On auto-eroticism in its relations with narcissism", *French Journal of Psychoanalysis*, No. 5-6.
COSNIER J. (1987), *Vicissitudes of Femininity*, Paris, Puf.
COURNUT J. (1989), "The two anti-cathexes" *New Journal of Psychoanalysis*, No. 39.
DE M'UZAN M. (1977), *A Case of Perverse Masochism*, Paris, Gallimard.
DELASSUS J.-M. (2001), *The Genius of the Foetus*, Paris, Dunod.
DICK P.K. (1979), "Recall Mechanism", in *The Golden Age of Science Fiction*, Paris, Pocket.
FAIN M. (1992), "Operative life and the traumatic neurosis potential", *French Journal of Psychoanalysis*, No. 2.
FAIN M., "On hypochondria", *Papers of the Centre for Psychoanalysis and Psychotherapy*, No. 21.
FEDIDA J. (1985), "Diurnal residues, life residues", Symposium "Life events and psychopathology", Simep.
FERENCZI S., *Complete Works* (4 vol.), Payot, 1977.
FERENCZI S. (1932), *Clinical Journal*, Paris, Payot, 1990.
FERRO A. (2000), *Psychoanalysis as an Open Book*, Toulouse, Eres.
FINE A. (1992), "Regression as organiser", *French Journal of Psychoanalysis*, No. 4.
FREUD S. (1883), *Letters*, Paris, Gallimard, 1979
FREUD S. (1890-1920), *Results, Ideas, Problems*, Jean Laplanche edition, vol. 1, Paris, Puf, Library of Psychoanalysis, 1991
FREUD S. (1895*a*), "Outline of a scientific psychology, in *Birth of Psychoanalysis*, Paris, Puf, 1950
FREUD S. (1895*b*), "Manuscript G" in "Letters to Fliess", in *Birth of Psychoanalysis*, Paris, Puf, 1950
FREUD S. (1895*c*), *Birth of Psychoanalysis*, Paris, Puf, 1950
FREUD S., BREUER G. (1895*c*), *Studies on Hysteria*, Paris, Puf (1975)
FREUD S. (1899), "The aetiology of hysteria", in *Neurosis, Psychosis and Perversion*, Paris, Puf, 1973
FREUD S. (1899), "Screen memories", in *Neurosis, Psychosis and Perversion*, Paris, Puf, 1973
FREUD S. (1900), *The Interpretation of Dreams*, Paris, Puf, 1973

FREUD S. (1901), *The Psychopathology of Everyday Life*, Paris, Puf, 1997
FREUD S. (1905*a*), *Three Essays on the Theory of Sexuality*, Paris, Gallimard, 1987
FREUD S. (1905*b*), "Fragments of an analysis of a case of hysteria (Dora)", in *Five Psychoanalyses*, Paris, Puf, 1970
FREUD S. (1907), *The Man with the Rats: Journal of an Analysis*, Paris, Puf, 2000
FREUD S. (1911*a*), "The two principles of mental functioning", in *Results, Ideas, Problems*, No. 1, Paris, Puf, 1984
FREUD S. (1912), "Contributions to a discussion on masturbation", in *Results, Ideas, Problems*, No. 1, Paris, Puf, 1984
FREUD S. (1914), "On narcissism: an introduction", in *Sexual Life*, Paris, Puf, 1969
FREUD S. (1915*a*), "Repression", in *Metapsychologies*, Paris, Gallimard, 1940
FREUD S. (1915*b*), "Instincts and their vicissitudes", in *Metapsychologies*, Paris, Gallimard, Coll. Ideas 1940
FREUD S. (1916), *Introductory Lectures*, Paris, Petite Bibliothèque Payot, 1969
FREUD S. (1917), "Mourning and melancholia", in *Metapsychologies*, Paris, Gallimard, Coll. Ideas, 1940
FREUD S. (1918), "Wolf Man", in *Five Psychoanalyses*, Paris, Puf, 1970
FREUD S. (1919), "The uncanny", Paris, Gallimard, 1985
FREUD S. (1919), "A child is being beaten", in *Neurosis, Psychosis and Perversion*, Paris, Puf, 1973
FREUD S. (1920), *Beyond the Pleasure Principle*, Paris, Payot, 1982
FREUD S. (1923), "The Ego and the Id", in *Essays on Psychoanalysis*, Petite Bibliothèque Payot, 1982
FREUD S. (1924), "The economic problem of masochism", in *Neurosis, Psychosis and Perversion*, Paris, Puf, 1973
FREUD S. (1926), *Inhibition, Symptom and Anxiety*, Paris, Puf, 1968
FREUD S. (1927), "Fetishism", in *Sexual Life*, Paris, Puf, 1969
FREUD S. (1929), *Civilisation and its Discontents*, Paris, Puf, 1971
FREUD S. (1936), "A disturbance of memory on the Acropolis", in *Results, Ideas, Problems*, No. 2, Paris, Puf, 1985
FREUD S. (1937*a*), "Analysis terminable and interminable", in *Results, Ideas, Problems*, No. 2, Paris, Puf, 1985

FREUD S. (1937*b*), "Constructions in Analysis", in *Results, Ideas, Problems*, No. 2, Paris, Puf, 1985
FREUD S. (1937*c*), "The split in the ego, translation" in *Results, Ideas, Problems*, No. 2, Paris, Puf, 1985
FREUD S. (1938), *Psychoanalysis Digest*, Paris, Puf, 1978
FREUD S. (1939), *Moses and Monotheism*, Paris, Gallimard, 1986
GAMMIL J. (1989), "Reflections on contraphobic mechanisms and the depressive position", *French Journal of Psychoanalysis*, No. 3.
GIBEAULT A. (1995), "Hypochondria", *French Journal of Psychoanalysis Monograph.*
GREEN A. (1973), *Vibrant Discourse*, Paris, Puf
GREEN A. (1990), "Why pain", in *Private Madness*, NRF Gallimard
GREEN A. (2002), *Clinical Thought*, Paris, Odile Jacob
GUILLAUMIN J. (1983), *The Psyche*, Paris, Puf
GUILLAUMIN J. (1996), "The loss object in Freud's thought", in *The Object*, Le Bouscat (Gironde), Spirit of the Age
GUILLAUMIN J. (2000), *The Invention of the Death Instinct*, Paris, Dunod
GUILLAUMIN J. (2001), "The Image between the inside and the outside" *French Journal of Psychoanalysis*, "Figurability", No. 4.
HOCHMANN J. (1992), "The autoerotic foundations of thinking", Conference at Paris Psychoanalytical Society.
HOCHMANN J. (2001), "Institution and Narration", Conference at Nîmes, October.
JAMES H. (1963), "The Beast in the Jungle", in *The Pupil and Other Stories*, Paris, 10-18, 1996
JEAMMET PH. (2000), *The Enigma of Masochism*, Paris, Puf
JEANNEAU A. (1985), "Hysteria", *French Journal of Psychoanalysis*, No. 1.
JONES E. (1969), *Sigmund Freud: Life and Work*, vol. 1, 2 and 3, Paris, Puf
KHAN M. (1974), "The resentment of the hysteric", in *New Journal of Psychoanalysis*, No. 10
LAPLANCHE J. (1970), *Life and Death in Psychoanalysis*, Paris, Flammarion
LAPLANCHE J., PONTALIS J.-B. (1967), *Vocabulary of Psychoanalysis*, Paris, Puf
LE BRETON D. (2002), *Identity Signs: Tattoos, Piercings and Other Body Marks*, Paris, ed. Metailié

LECLAIRE S. (1975), *A Child is being Killed*, Paris, Seuil, The Freudian Field
LEVI P. (1957), *If This is a Man*, Paris, Juillard
LEVY F. (1988), *Crossfire: From Hypochondriac to Doctor Despite Himself*, Meyzieu (Rhône), Caesura
LUBTCHANSKY J. (1973), "The economic point of view in hysteria, from the concept of trauma", in *French Journal of Psychoanalysis*, No. 3.
MARTY P., M'UZAN M. DE, DAVID CH. (1963), *Psychosomatic Investigation*, Paris, Puf
McDOUGALL J. (1982), *The Theatre of the Mind*, Paris, Gallimard
MERSKEY H. (1979), Journal "Pain" (1979-6), pp. 49-252
MILLER P. (1999), "Pain, a survival therapy", *French Journal of Psychoanalysis*, No. 15.
NERVAL G. DE (1854), "Anteros" in *Chimera*, La Pléiade, vol. 1, 1989
OBADIA J.-P. (1990), "When the birth of a masochistic perversion takes over from a serious somatic disorder", *French Journal of Psychoanalysis*, No. 3.
ODDY M. (1999), "The Freudian concept of extreme representation", *French Journal of Psychoanalysis*, No. 5.
PERRIER F. (1959), "Psychoanalysis of the hypochondriac", in *Rue de la Chaussée d'Antin*, Paris, Albin Michel, 1994
POE E.A. (1841), "A Descent into the Maelstrom" in *Prose Works*, Paris, Gallimard, Bibliothèque de la Pléiade (1951)
PONTALIS J.-B. (1977), *Between the Dream and Psychic Pain*, Paris, Gallimard
PONTALIS J.-B. (1988), *Losing Sight*, Paris, Gallimard
RAFFALLI B. (1987), Preface to *Remembrance of Things Past*, Proust, ed. R. Laffont, Bouquins, vol. 2 and 3
RICOEUR P. (1983), *Time and Narrative*, Paris, Seuil
ROLLAND J.-C. (1986), "A torture victim", *New Journal of Psychoanalysis*, No. 33.
ROSE D. (1997), *Primal Endurance*, Paris, Puf, Coll. The Red Line
ROSENBERG B. (1991), "Fatal masochism, lifesaving masochism", in *French Journal of Psychoanalysis Monograph*
ROSOLATO G. (1978), *The Unknown Relationship*, Paris, Gallimard
ROUX M.-L. (1984), "Affected and disaffected bodies", *French Journal of Psychoanalysis*, No. 6.
SCHILDER P. (1968), *Body Image*, Paris, Gallimard

SCHNEIDER M. (1980), *Memory Wounds*, Paris, Gallimard
SCHUR M. (1975), *Freud: Living and Dying*, Paris, Gallimard
SMADJA Cl. (1997), "Unthinkable pain" in *Disquiet: Anxiety and Violence* (ed. J. Cournut), Paris, Puf
SMADJA Cl. (1999), "The enigma of pain in essential depression", *French Journal of Psychoanalysis*, No. 15.
STOLLER R.J. (1991), "XSM", *New Journal of Psychoanalysis*, "Excess", No. 43
SZWEC G. (1996), "Erotic subversion and self-calming subversion", in *French Psychosomatic Journal*, No. 10.
SZWEC G. (1998), "Life, directions for use", in *French Journal of Psychoanalysis*, No. 5.
WINNICOTT D. (1982), "Fear of breakdown", in *Essays on Psychoanalysis*, Paris, Petite Bibliothèque Payot

INDEX